KATHLEEN LYNN

For Ciarán

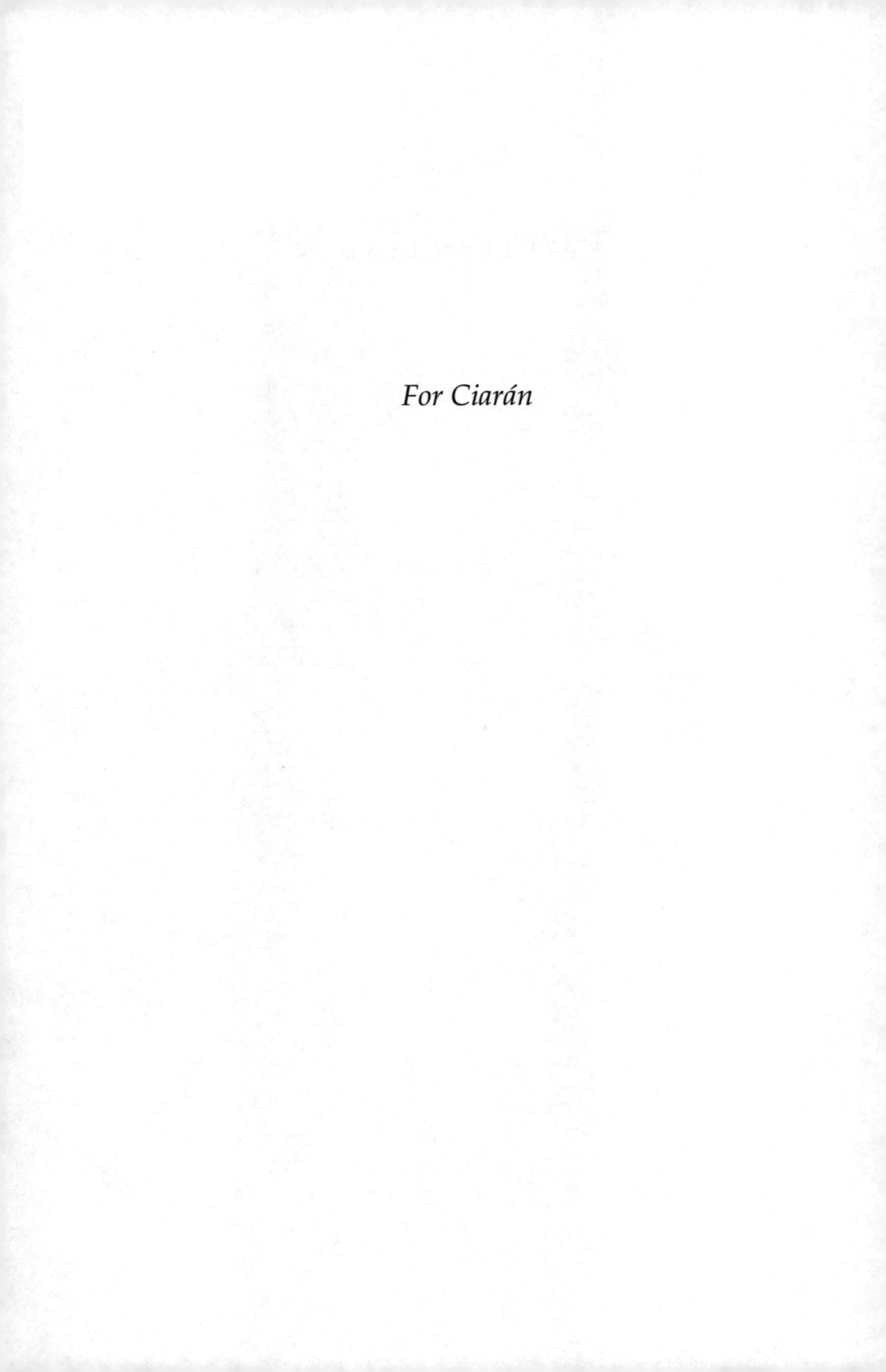

KATHLEEN LYNN
Irishwoman, Patriot, Doctor

MARGARET Ó HÓGARTAIGH
Victoria University of Wellington

IRISH ACADEMIC PRESS
DUBLIN • PORTLAND, OR

First published in 2006 by
IRISH ACADEMIC PRESS
44, Northumberland Road, Dublin 4, Ireland

and in the United States of America by
IRISH ACADEMIC PRESS
c/o ISBS, Suite 300, 920 NE 58th Avenue
Portland, Oregon 97213–3644

© 2006 Margaret Ó hÓgartaigh

WEBSITE: www.iap.ie

British Library Cataloguing in Publication Data
A catalogue entry is available on request

10–digit ISBN 0–7165–2842–8 (hbk)
13–digit ISBN 978–0–7165–2842–5
10–digit ISBN 0–7165–2843–6 (pbk)
13–digit ISBN 978–0–7165–2843–2

Library of Congress Cataloging-in-Publication Data
An entry can be found on request

All rights reserved. Without limiting the rights under copyright reserved alone, no part of this publication may be reproduced, stored in or introduced into a retrieval system, or transmitted, in any form or by any means (electronic, mechanical, photocopying, recording or otherwise), without the prior written permission of both the copyright owner and the above publisher of this book.

Typeset by Carrigboy Typesetting Services, County Cork.
Printed by Antony Rowe Ltd, Chippenham, Wiltshire.

Contents

List of illustrations	vi
Acknowledgements	vii
Introduction	1
CHAPTER ONE The making of a female doctor, 1874–1911	6
CHAPTER TWO Rebellious womanhood, 1912–30	18
CHAPTER THREE 'A University for Mothers', 1919–30	64
CHAPTER FOUR The politics of children's health, 1928–39	92
CHAPTER FIVE A servant of the nation, 1940–55	119
CHAPTER SIX Radical witness	146
Bibliography	158
Index	176

List of illustrations

1. Dr Kathleen Lynn and Madeleine ffrench-Mullen, *circa*, 1919. (*St. Ultan's Annual Report, 1945,* Courtesy of the Royal College of Physicians of Ireland).

2. Dr. Kathleen Lynn, Arthur Griffith, Éamon de Valera and Michael Collins, 1921. (Courtesy of the Royal College of Physicians of Ireland).

3. Dream Hospital, what St. Ultan's might have been, *circa* 1936. (*St. Ultan's Annual Report, 1945,* Courtesy of the Royal College of Physicians of Ireland).

4. St. Ultan's Annual General Meeting, 1944, Dr. Kathleen Lynn, Dr. Thomas Gillman Moorhead, Dr. Dorothy Stopford Price and Sister Mulligan, the Matron). (*St. Ultan's Annual Report, 1945,* Courtesy of the Royal College of Physicians of Ireland).

5. Dr. Kathleen Lynn and St. Ultan's patient with Oxygen Hood, with Rathmines Junior Red Cross and a nurse, 1948. (Courtesy of the Royal College of Physicians of Ireland).

6. Child on stroller, possibly a polio victim, with Dr. Kathleen Lynn, 1950. (Courtesy of the Royal College of Physicians of Ireland).

7. Child on a rocking horse with Dr. Lynn, a nurse and Rathmines Junior Red Cross, 1954. (Courtesy of the Royal College of Physicians of Ireland).

8. Postgraduate Course Participants and Staff of St. Ultan's, 1949. (Courtesy of the Royal College of Physicians of Ireland).

Acknowledgements

My thanks to Maria Luddy, who asked me to write a biography of Lynn. Her patience is much appreciated. Without her, this biography would never have been written. Lisa Hyde was a perfect editor, patient, perceptive and professional. I would also like to thank my Irish Academic Press reader for astute advice and my copy editor for reading my work so carefully. Most of this book was written while teaching in St. Patrick's College, Drumcondra. I am particularly grateful to Pauric Travers, who engendered a creative, co-operative and caring working environment. I would also like to thank Jimmy Kelly, whose industry was inspirational; Dáire Keogh and Carla King, both constant supporters, and Marian Lyons, whose professionalism and encouragement are appreciated. Other friends in St. Patrick's, Gearoidín Uí Laighleis, Cora Cregan, Alan Titley, Ruth McManus, Máirín Nic Eoin, Olivia Bree, Matthew Stout, Aida Keane and Fionnuala Waldron have all endured my wayward woes with Lynn.

The Contemporary Irish History Seminar at Trinity College Dublin has proved to be enormously stimulating and its accessibility is a model for other seminars. I would like to thank Louis Cullen and Eunan O'Halpin for their support. Finola Kennedy's and Margaret MacCurtain's constant encouragement and wise advice are greatly appreciated. Caitriona Clear and Joe Lee were engaging and enlightening. My thanks to Marie Coleman, Anne Dolan, William Murphy, Gillian O'Brien and Diarmuid Whelan who were always on the look-out for Lynn. David Murphy was a wonderful fount of wit and wisdom. Lindsey Earner-Byrne's original and path-breaking work on motherhood enlightened me and we have shared many pleasurable moments discussing history. Her characteristically insightful comments on my work are much appreciated. Greta Jones' work on the history of medicine is inspirational. Séamus Mac Gabhann, editor of *Ríocht na Midhe*, was supportive and I have learned much from his astute editing.

Guy Beiner, Angela Bourke, Ciara Breathnach, Anna Brioscú, the late Frances Carruthers, Jack and Tom Curran, Mairéad Dunlevy, Martina Farren, David Fitzpatrick, Roy Foster, Tom Garvin, Brian Hanley, the late Ursula Hurley, Alvin Jackson, Michael Kennedy, Rita Lees, John Logan, Murdina MacFarquhar-Desmond, Mary Teresa Moran, Sinéad McCoole, Fearghal McGarry, Ellen More, Ailish O'Brien, Andrew O'Brien, Anne O'Connor, Katherine O'Donnell, Daithí Ó Corráin, Cormac Ó Gráda, Séamus Ó Maitiú, Rebecca Pelan, Rosemary Raughter, Susannah Riordan, Medb Ruane, Matt Russell, Vanessa Rutherford, Rob Somerville-Woodward, Conor Ward, Sinéad Walsh, Kerry 'Ciotóg' Wardick and the late William Wynne helped me in various ways.

Research in the United States for this biography was greatly aided by the award of a Fulbright Fellowship. Kevin Whelan characteristically provided me with useful leads in Boston College. He even drew a map. Furthermore, the Irish Studies centre at Connolly House provided the perfect environment for an interdisciplinary approach. In particular, Seamus Connolly, Cathy McLoughlin, Rob Savage and Peg Preston provided much stimulation and made me feel so welcome. Peg has alerted me to various sources and has always been extremely supportive. I am grateful to Kevin O'Neill who asked me to teach a course on Irish women in medicine. My students, Lia Parico, Christina Price, Teresa Immediata, Liz Holland, Meghan Kane and Jillian Lo Piano have all provided me with new insights and ideas. Nadia Smith has also stimulated me with her innovative work. Further afield, Lynn's direct descendants in Australia, particularly Lenore McKay, have been most helpful and generous with sources.

As usual, I am indebted to archivists and librarians. Robert Mills, librarian at the Royal College of Physicians, is a researcher's dream. He constantly provided the sources for my many requests and his impressive knowledge of the history of medicine made my research all the more rewarding. The St. Ultan's papers have found a happy home in his care. Furthermore, I would like to thank the Royal College of Physicians in Ireland for supporting the transcription of Kathleen Lynn's voluminous diaries. Margaret

Acknowledgements

Connolly's meticulous work has made Lynn more accessible. Mary O'Doherty, archivist at the Royal College of Surgeons, was always a fount of information. David Sheehy, archivist at the Dublin Diocesan Archives, regularly alerted me to important documents and was a mine of information on Irish history. Fergus O'Farrell, Tim Lyne and Geraldine Breen facilitated my access to the important Adelaide Hospital archives. Patrick Sweeney, Gerry Long, Gerry Lyne, Colette O'Daly, Ciarán McEniry, Colette O'Flaherty, Francis Carroll, Patrick Sweeney, Tom Desmond, Jim Dunne, James Harte, Sophie O'Brien, Jimmy Dunne, Sandra McDermott and Jimmy Flemming of the National Library of Ireland have been most helpful. Aisling Lockhart, Jane Maxwell and Ursula Mitchel of the TCD Manuscripts Departments, where the important Dorothy Stopford Price papers are located, were obliging, as were Seamus Helferty, Lisa Collins and Kate Manning of the UCD archives department. Caitriona Crowe and all the staff at the National Archives endured my obscure requests for information and always managed to find my files. Alan Manning, Pat Brennan, Chris Donovan and Victor Laing at the Military Archives and all the staff at the Donal Cregan Library, St. Patrick's College, Drumcondra (especially Molly Sheehan, at inter-library loans) were helpful and encouraging. Norma Jessop of UCD Special Collections located significant sources. Bernie Cunningham of the Royal Irish Academy has been a great guide and I have benefited from her bibliographical gifts. Her colleague, Pauric Dempsey, located important sources for me in the Academy's library. The Dictionary of Irish Biography staff, especially James McGuire, R.A.J. Hawkins, Cathy Hayes, Jim Quinn and Frances Clarke provided useful information. Bríd Leahy and Mary Clark at the Dublin City Archives were most helpful. Alison Duck and Noelle Dowling at the Brother Allen Library, O'Connell Schools were enormously helpful and their 1916 material was invaluable.

In the United States, Martha Stone, librarian at the Treadwell Library and Jeffrey Mifflin, curator of Special Collections, at Massachusetts General Hospital, and Mary Moriarity at St. John's Seminary Library in Boston were helpful in tracking down sources. Kathy Williams and Daniel Carey at the O'Neill Library in Boston College greatly facilitated my researches. Doris Ann Sweet of the

Countway Medical Library, Harvard University was most obliging. Ellen Shea, the reference librarian, at the Schlesinger library at the Radcliffe Institute for Advanced Study, Harvard University, answered my queries with clarity and precision; her colleague Kathy Herrlich was equally helpful. Milissa Boyer Kafes, archivist at the Rockefeller Archive Center, kindly sent me valuable material and made my visit to the archives all the more productive. My thanks to all the helpful staff at Melrose Public Library. Melrose Running Club members were always enthusiastic and supportive. Brendan, Carol, Delaney and Cameret Bannister were wonderful hosts in Melrose.

I have learned much from the History Section of the Royal Academy of Medicine in Ireland. In particular, contemporaries of Lynn and medical practitioners, such as Rosarie Barry, Alan Browne, Davis Coakley, John Fleetwood, Peter Froggatt, Peter Gatenby, Jack Lyons, Livinia Meenan, Pauline O'Connell, Liam Ó Sé and Barbara Stokes have all shared their knowledge with me. It was a pleasure to learn from their professional experiences in paediatrics and public health. The late Joe Robins will be greatly missed and he cheerfully shared his detailed knowledge of public health. The Medical Council at Lynn House was supportive and encouraging, particularly its president John Hillery, and the registrar, John Lamont. Thanks also to Lisa Molloy.

The vibrant Rathmines, Ranelagh and Rathgar Historical Association and Charlemont Clinic facilitated my work in so many ways; my thanks to Angela O'Connell, Noel Healy, Tom Harris and the late Deirdre Kelly. Rathmines resident and descendant of Countess Plunkett, Honor Ó Brolcháin, kindly gave me a guided tour of Lynn's former residence at 9 Belgrave Road. Her interest and knowledge greatly assisted my research. My sincere thanks to Colum, 'professor of camogie', King, Peter, 'I would never throw a hurley on my head', Dowd and Keith, keep smiling, Heffernan, as well as all the 'girls' (aged 45 and under!) at Ráth Tó Camogie Club for their diligence and enthusiasm. Thanks to Peter Doherty, of Ratoath Dental Centre, whose care and compassion, as well as his professional gifts, ensured that this book was completed pain free.

My father has encouraged me for as long as I can remember. My mother, who died before I began this book, would have liked to

Acknowledgements

read it. My siblings, Anne Marie, Eveleen, Jean, Teresa, Emer, James and Brian facilitated my work in different ways. I am grateful to Eimear, Proinséas and the late Seosamh Ó hÓgartaigh, for their kindness and hospitality. My greatest debt, as usual, is to my husband Ciarán. He never complained and even seemed to enjoy the ménage à trois in Massachusetts and Meath.

MARGARET Ó HÓGARTAIGH
Ráth Tó and Wellington
July 2006

Introduction

A BIOGRAPHY OF Dr Kathleen Lynn (1874–1955) is long overdue. A staunch republican and committed member of the Church of Ireland, she defied her family's unionist politics. However, Lynn remained faithful to her family. Two strands – the poverty of so many people, and political activity, which sought to eliminate the causes of that poverty – were to be continually intertwined in Dr Lynn's career. Born in County Mayo prior to the establishment of the Land League, Lynn died in Dublin three decades after the independent Irish state was established. In many senses, her life mirrors the numerous changes that took place in Ireland during these eighty years. During her lifetime, women gained access to higher education and the professions and Lynn was to benefit from the revolution in women's education in the late nineteenth century.[1] When the independent Irish state was established in the 1920s, Lynn endured the restrictions imposed by reactionary revolutionaries. She was part of a generation that cut its political teeth in the heady days of the late nineteenth and early twentieth centuries. Her activism in the cause of suffrage, as well as involvement in the 1916 Rising, and national politics in the 1920s, ensured her political prominence. However, like many, Lynn became dissatisfied with the slow rate of change in subsequent decades.

Lynn's popular and professional reputation rests on her medical work on behalf of the Dublin poor. Such was her fame, even in her lifetime, that one Dublin woman was christened Kathleen Lynn.[2] In 1997 the Medical Council decided to name its central office Lynn House.[3] Appropriately, it is located between her home in Rathmines and St Ultan's Hospital for Infants, which she co-founded in 1919, on Charlemont Street. Lynn believed in the political philosophy of Theobald Wolfe Tone and James Connolly, and their republicanism, and social radicalism informed her medical activism. Tone is seen as the father of Irish republicanism while Connolly's socialism inspired Lynn in the years leading up to the 1916 Rising and thereafter. Lynn admired both men. She was a regular visitor to the grave of Tone in Bodenstown, while Connolly's writings on nationalism and socialism clearly influenced her thinking. Intriguingly, it was the problematic Helena Molony, highly strung, yet charismatic, and eventually alcoholic, who introduced Lynn to socialism and nationalism in the 1910s.[4]

Lynn was a pioneering paediatrician. In many senses, the neglect of Lynn is part of a wider historiographical neglect of socio-medical history. Lynn believed that the future citizens of the nation were frequently neglected. Her life was devoted to others, yet she was not someone to be trifled with. This biography will trace her career from comfortable beginnings to socialist commitment. Her pragmatic socialism found practical expression in St Ultan's Hospital for Infants. She remained devoted to the hospital until her death in 1955. Lynn's career was preoccupied with timeless themes, the care of children and the limits of revolutions.

How significant a figure is Kathleen Lynn in Irish history?[5] J. J. Lee in his influential textbook, *Ireland, 1912–1985*, mentions Lynn's 'indignant response' to the allegations that the 'learned ladies' in the National University Women Graduates' Association were absent from the struggle for national independence.[6] Lynn, as Irene Finn correctly suggests, is better known as a rebel than as a doctor. Her prominence in the 1916 Rising ensures her fame, but she was also a radical woman in a conservative and male-dominated profession.[7] Lynn's generation saw the conservatism of the Irish Free State as a violation of the work of the revolutionary activists of the 1910s.

This biography will argue that while her political radicalism is undeniable, Lynn's most radical contribution was in medicine. Works on the history of medicine in Ireland, not surprisingly, acknowledge her activities. She emerges as an 'evocative' name in Peter Froggatt's careful analysis of medical schools in Ireland,[8] while J. B. Lyons is at pains to claim that she was 'basically a pacifist'.[9] Women like Lynn used their political experience and considerable energy to fight for the unheard voices in Irish history; children, the urban poor and women with large families.

Introduction

Lynn's professional and social activities were possible because she had a good income. Furthermore, she could sustain others both economically and emotionally. Her many trips, undertaken for political and medical reasons, would not have been possible if she had not had a professional career. Her socio-economic background, as the daughter of a Church of Ireland canon, made a medical career possible. Most people of her generation, and for many generations afterwards, were educated at first level only. She was fortunate, in both senses, to be a member of a social class which could afford the extensive education associated with a medical career. Despite these social advantages, she was not to enjoy the full fruits of her labours.

How did Lynn survive the various vicissitudes of her life? Clearly her relationship with Madeleine ffrench-Mullen, 'dearest MffM.' sustained her.[10] They lived together for thirty years until ffrench-Mullen's death in 1944.[11] Ffrench-Mullen was Lynn's closest confidante. The eldest daughter of a naval doctor, she was born in Malta in 1880. She attended the Sacred Heart Convent at Leeson Street in Dublin between 1892 and 1898. Her father was an 'ardent Home Ruler', according to Hanna Sheehy Skeffington. Local elections in Dundrum, where the family lived after her father's retirement, ensured that Madeleine was 'plunged into politics, [with] her father eagerly instructing her.' His death, when ffrench-Mullen's younger sister Pearl was still a baby, left the eldest with many responsibilities since her mother was in poor health. The family spent a lot of time on the continent and ffrench-Mullen was in Belgium when the First World War began.[12] They moved to Ireland in 1914. Having seen Lynn give a first aid lecture at Sinn Féin headquarters, ffrench-Mullen met her at Stradbrook Hall where she was caring for Belgian refugees. Ffrench-Mullen's interest in children was evident early on as she edited the 'Children's Corner' for *Bean na hÉireann*.[13]

Maeve Carroll, a neighbour, was intrigued by these two women. They 'wore collars and ties and hats like men's and rode three-wheeled bicycles exactly like a child's tricycle.'[14] At some stage, according to Archbishop Donal Caird, a friend of Lynn, ffrench-Mullen had a leg amputated. Perhaps this explains the unusual mode of transport! At the first anniversary of ffrench-Mullen's death in 1945, Lynn remembered how her great friend 'nestled down, close to me while I sat beside her with her head on my shoulder'.[15] The importance of friendships is one of the under-explored areas of Irish history. While there is no evidence of sexual activity between Lynn and ffrench-Mullen, clearly they were very intimate. Furthermore, Lynn kept a vast amount of ffrench-Mullen material which she donated, in the late 1940s, to Brother Allen for his 1916 collection, at the Christian Brothers Archive, O'Connell Schools, Dublin. This material includes an affectionate letter to Lynn from the British suffragist, Sylvia Pankhurst, which has lain undisturbed for many years.[16] Pankhurst thought Lynn 'must be lonely' without ffrench-Mullen. Did Lynn's sense of humour prompt her to give this material to a Christian Brother who was fascinated by 1916?

Lynn, like other women, was to be politically marginalised in the late 1920s. She remained a committed republican. Her life deserves examination for the light it throws on a forgotten generation of women who seemed to hold so much promise in the early years of the new state. Their later lives can be traced through rarely read documentation in archives and libraries. Revd William Wynne's decision to donate his relative's diaries to the Royal College of Physicians in Ireland has made this biography possible. Lynn's voluminous diaries, over half a million words, are both revealing and immediate. They are a veritable 'who was who' in Irish nationalist life. She began her diary on 16 March 1916 and the last entry is dated 25 April 1955. The diary was a therapeutic escape from the frustrations of everyday toil. It was 'a spiritual account book'.[17] Occasionally it bristles with frustration. However, it was also Lynn's way of reassuring herself that her life's work was not in vain. Only by carefully assessing all her activities can we even attempt to understand this fascinating and multi-faceted woman.

NOTES

1 See Mary Cullen (ed.), *Girls Don't Do Honours: Irish Women and Education in the Nineteenth and Twentieth Centuries* (Dublin, 1987).
2 I am grateful to Eilís Ní Bhrádaigh for pointing out to me that Kathleen Lynn Fullerton was named after Lynn in the 1920s.

Introduction

3 Comhairle na nDochtúirí Leighis/Medical Council *Newsletter*, June 1997. I am grateful to Mary O'Doherty, archivist, Royal College of Surgeons, for bringing this newsletter to my attention. The Adelaide and Meath Hospitals incorporating the National Children's Hospital (Tallaght Hospital) also has a ward named after Kathleen Lynn.
4 Nell Regan, 'Helena Molony (1883–1967)' in Mary Cullen and Maria Luddy (eds), *Female Activists: Irish Women and Change, 1900–1960* (Dublin, 2001), pp. 141–68.
5 Lynn features in Roddy Day, Fionnuala Waldron, Tommy Maher and Pauric Travers, *Time Traveller 1* (Dublin, 1996), pp. 72–3. This history book is recommended for eight/nine year olds.
6 J. J. Lee, *Ireland, 1912–1985, Politics and Society* (Cambridge, 1989), p. 207.
7 Irene Finn, 'Women in the medical profession in Ireland, 1876–1919', in Bernadette Whelan (ed.), *Women and Paid Work in Ireland, 1500–1930* (Dublin, 2000), pp. 102–19, p. 118.
8 Peter Froggatt, 'Competing Philosophies: the "Preparatory" Medical Schools of the Royal Belfast Academical Institution and the Catholic University of Ireland, 1835–1909', in Greta Jones and Elizabeth Malcolm (eds), *Medicine, Disease and the State in Ireland, 1650–1940* (Cork, 1999), pp. 59–84, p. 77.
9 J. B. Lyons, *Brief Lives of Irish Doctors* (Dublin, 1978), pp. 159–60, p. 160.
10 Lynn Diaries (hereafter LD) 6 June 1944. These diaries are located in the Royal College of Physicians in Ireland (RCPI) Dublin. They have been carefully transcribed by Margaret Connolly under the auspices of the RCPI. They were donated to the RCPI by William Wynne, a relative of Lynn.
11 Lynn's first witness statement, Allen Library, Dublin.
12 The Madeleine ffrench-Mullen file in the Allen Library includes many postcards to ffrench-Mullen in Belguim in 1913–14. Her father, who was originally from Tuam, was an unsuccessful Parnellite candidate in South Dublin in the 1892 election; obituary of Douglas ffrench-Mullen, ffrench-Mullen's uncle, 17 April 1920, in *British Medical Journal*, Kirkpatrick Biographical Archive, RCPI.
13 H.S.S., [Hanna Sheehy Skeffington] 'In Memoriam Madeleine ffrench Mullen', in *St Ultan's Annual Report*, 1945, pp. 13–18. *Bean na hÉireann* was the organ of the nationalist women in Inghínídhe na hÉireann.
14 Maeve Carroll, 'The Rebel Road – childhood memories of "The Troubles"', *Irish Times*, 24 June 1970.
15 LD, 25 May 1945.
16 Pankhurst to Lynn, 7 December 1916, in ffrench-Mullen file, Allen Library, Dublin.
17 Alvin Jackson, 'J.C. Beckett: politics, faith, scholarship', in *Irish Historical Studies*, vol. xxxiii, no. 130, Nov., 2002, pp. 129–50, p. 129

CHAPTER ONE

The making of a female doctor, 1874–1911

KATHLEEN FLORENCE LYNN was born on 28 January 1874 in Mullaghfarry, two miles from Killala in north Mayo. She was the second oldest child of Reverend Robert Lynn, then a Church of Ireland clergyman in Killaney near Killala and later a canon at Cong, and Catherine Wynne, the daughter of Reverend Richard Wynne of Drumcliffe, County Sligo.[1] Lynn's elder sister Nan had been born a year earlier and the family was completed by two younger siblings, John and Muriel. Lynn's maternal grandfather was a younger son of Owen Wynne, a Member of Parliament for the English constituency of Hazelwood, and Anne Maxwell, the Earl of Farnham's sister. Despite this slight aristocratic connection, Lynn did not associate herself with the privileged, and her later career was primarily concerned with those in need.

Mayo in the 1870s experienced significant poverty, though Lynn would have been insulated, to a certain extent, from the near-famine conditions of the late 1870s.[2] Interestingly, both the Wynnes and the Lynns were noted for their philanthropy. It is clear from her diaries that Lynn was devoted to her mother. Middle-class women, including clergymen's wives, such as Catherine Wynne, were often involved in philanthropic activity. Over twenty years after her mother's death, Lynn wrote that an old friend, Bessie McQuiade, 'spoke of dear Mother, as always, no one could go to Cong & not be better for seeing her, so true.'[3] Her mother's kindness must have been an important influence for Lynn. The poor of Mayo endured illness and disease which were intensified and exacerbated by limited medical facilities.

Furthermore, the suffering caused by the bad economic conditions of the late 1870s stimulated intense political activity, including the establishment of the Land League, which sought to improve the lot of tenant farmers. These two themes, poverty and political activity, particularly that which sought to eliminate the causes of that poverty, were to be continually intertwined in Lynn's professional career. Lynn's Mayo childhood may have introduced her to the radicalism of Michael Davitt and the Land League. However, Lynn, like many from middle-class backgrounds, wanted to help the poor on her own terms, and she would decide what was best for them. Given the poverty and social deprivation, it is not surprising that doctors held positions of particular importance and influence. Hence, Lynn's early years in the west of Ireland undoubtedly helped to shape her perspectives. Moreover, the Land League may have given the young Lynn her first glimpse of female political protest. Donald Jordan has suggested that as an 'open, constitutional mass movement, the Land War provided opportunities for women to participate. Its open-air meetings were open to all, with women often attending in large numbers'.[4] Janet Te Brake has gone even further in her analysis of peasant protest during the Land League years. She suggests that involvement in the Land League (particularly the Ladies' Land League) ensured that women were 'active rather than passive' in rural revolts.[5] Lynn lived during a period of radical social and economic change, and land agitation provided women with the opportunity to play an active role in a political organisation. Furthermore, charitable activity, including the provision of charity to evicted families, gave middle-class women a public role during this period. It was a role which would be extended by Lynn and others in the twentieth century, when political unrest disrupted families. Many would see philanthropy as apolitical, but it was a politicising experience.[6] Adrian Wilson has suggested that 'politics and charity were reciprocally related'.[7]

When Lynn was eight years old the family moved to Shrule in County Longford.[8] Lynn had a professional role model in nearby Ballymahon. Dr Francis Smartt worked there while Lynn lived in Shrule.[9] He was able to 'ease the distress' of the local people.[10] Smartt was also her first cousin.[11] Furthermore, Robert Lynn's father was a doctor, so Lynn had plenty of medical role models.

The family moved to Cong in 1882, when her father was appointed to the estate of the Guinness family. Lord Ardilaun experienced land agitation also and Lynn may have been aware of women defending their homes against eviction. The 'land agent of Sir Arthur Guinness was "doused with scalding water" by a young woman whose parents had recently been served with an eviction notice'.[12] Cong would have been quite a change for Lynn since it was often used as an aristocratic retreat and, in later years, she was apt to reminisce about the Prince of Wales' visit to Cong.[13] Her family's social standing ensured that they were invited to these aristocratic gatherings. Meanwhile, in wider society social tensions and conflict between landlords and tenant farmers persisted. As the daughter of a Church of Ireland clergyman, Lynn would have enjoyed the comforts of the manse, but, like all women, whether wealthy or poor, she did not enjoy any formal political power. The origins of women's overt political activity lay in the nineteenth century. In the same period, there was a quiet revolution in education.

Like many of her class, sex and generation, Lynn received tuition from a governess. There would have been an emphasis on languages. Furthermore, Lynn would have imbibed the spiritual atmosphere of the family home. She attended religious service daily. Lynn absorbed the climate of the late Victorian period with its emphasis on religious devotion and social reform.

Lynn was born into a middle-class, Protestant culture. The assurance of her background was surely largely responsible for her undoubted self confidence and ability to inspire and command others. The constraints of her time and sex imposed some limitations on her activities. Schooling was less of a priority for females, though Lynn was a member of the first generation of Irish women who benefited from changes in the educational system in the late nineteenth century. It remained a small minority (less than 10 per cent of the population) that proceeded beyond first-level education, but Kathleen Lynn was part of this important minority.

FORMAL EDUCATION

After her years with the governess in Cong, whom she simply categorised as 'good', Lynn received a more formal education in

Manchester and Dusseldorf.[14] She may have been sent to Dusseldorf because relatives, the Wynnes of Wicklow, had mining interests in Germany. Whatever the reason, Lynn became fluent in German and maintained her fluency throughout her long life. The extension of second-level education to females is one of the quiet revolutions of nineteenth-century Ireland. The choice of Alexandra College in Dublin for her second-level education was not surprising since it had established itself as an academically ambitious school, with a good reputation. Many of its graduates, primarily Protestant women, chose professional careers in medicine and education.[15] Her international educational experiences, as well as the progressive atmosphere at Alexandra College, gave her a cosmopolitan outlook and an interest in world affairs.

While Lynn was a student at Alexandra in the early 1890s, she would come under the influence of Isabella Mulvany, the headmistress. Mulvany emphasised academic subjects, hence students were prepared for paid employment. In a study of French education, Linda Clark points out that girls' education was not designed to 'prepare pupils for professional careers'; for example, the exclusion of Latin meant that women 'lacked an essential subject for baccalaureate and university entrance.'[16] Mulvany was insistent that girls take classical subjects and mathematics at Alexandra, and this was essential for Lynn if a medical career was being considered.

Furthermore, the 'cultural capital', amassed at Alexandra served Lynn well for the rest of her public life.[17] This intangible asset is difficult to define but it included art and musical appreciation. Cultural capital was accumulated during the extra-curricular activities that Alexandra encouraged. The university-like atmosphere of Alexandra, with its debating society which discussed current topics, undoubtedly engendered confidence amongst its students. It would surely have prepared Lynn and her contemporaries for public life. While attending Alexandra, Lynn studied arithmetic, geography, Latin, history and music as well as horticulture, and she enjoyed cycling and hockey.[18] The development of academic schools helped to pave the way for women's entrance into the universities. Several others of the first generation of medical women attended Alexandra, including Isabella Ovenden and Katherine Maguire. This, of course, is also a reflection on their socio-economic status, as the school catered primarily for the middle class. By 1918, in western Europe, only England, Wales and Norway had a higher percentage of females at second level than Ireland. More significantly, only Finland had a higher percentage of females at university.[19] Lynn's university career during the 1890s at the Catholic University Medical School occurred during a period of political and cultural vibrancy.

THE CATHOLIC UNIVERSITY MEDICAL SCHOOL

By the time Lynn began her medical studies in 1894, she was twenty years old. The general maturity of college students is consistent with American figures where only one-third of the female students at Stanford was aged less than twenty.[20] Students tended to be older because they began formal education later. By 1894, Lynn had studied in three different countries (Ireland, England and Germany) and was eager for further studies. Trinity College Dublin did not open its doors to women until 1904, and this primarily explains Lynn's arrival at the Catholic University Medical School in the 1890s. Given her denominational background, she would almost certainly have studied at Trinity had it been an option.

Significantly, women were admitted to Cecilia Street Medical School (subsequently the University College Dublin Medical School) before they could attend lectures at the Catholic University. Dr William Delaney, President of the Catholic University, or University College, between 1883 and 1888, was reluctant to accept female students.[21] Royal College of Science courses were taken as part of one's medical training. Katherine Maguire had taken botany and zoology courses at the Royal College of Science in 1887. She graduated with a first-class honours medical degree in 1891 and a Master's degree in medicine two years later.[22] She was Ireland's first female paediatrician. Lynn and Maguire later worked together in St Ultan's.

While opportunities were gradually opening up for women in medicine, some suggested that they should work in particular areas that were appropriate for the 'fairer sex'. Dr Sophia Jex-Blake,[23] who founded the London School of Medicine for Women in 1874, suggested that females should cater for female patients: 'perhaps we shall find the solution to some of our saddest social problems when educated and pure-minded women are brought more constantly in contact with their sinning and suffering sisters, in other relations as well as those of missionary effort'.[24] Lynn may have been influenced by these views and her career reinforced the perception that many women saw themselves as philanthropic professionals. However, this emphasis tended to define and confine female medical practitioners.

Lynn was a successful medical student. She enrolled at the Adelaide Hospital in October 1895.[25] She came first in practical anatomy in 1896, much to the delight of Alexandra College since this was 'a distinction not hitherto achieved by a woman'. Two years later, she was awarded the Barker Anatomical prize.[26] Students were expected to conduct their clinical training in various hospitals and the Adelaide was the most prominent Protestant hospital in Dublin. According to David Mitchell, Lynn applied for a residency in 1898 but was refused because of the absence of female accommodation.[27] Hence, she could not do her residency at the Adelaide. However, Lynn was able to obtain a residency at the Royal Victoria Eye and Ear Hospital, the 'first woman to do so',[28] and by October 1896 she was registered at Cecilia Street Medical School, where there were six females attending, only two of whom were Catholic. 'Professor Quinlan', according to F.O.C. Meenan, 'offered to surrender to the ladies his pharmacy laboratory and specimen room and these were fitted up as a waiting room and dissecting room for the use of the lady students'.[29] Obviously it was considered unacceptable for men and women to dissect in the same room! Lynn also gained valuable work experience in the National Maternity Hospital Holles Street, the Richmond Lunatic Asylum, and the Rotunda Lying-In Hospital, where she received a licentiate in midwifery.[30]

While women faced many difficulties in their professional careers, there were some male supporters within the educational system. Dr Ambrose Birmingham, Professor of Anatomy and Registrar of Cecilia Street, described female medical students in 1902 as 'hard-working, earnest and most conscientious'. Birmingham also noted that 'several ladies prefer to dissect in the general room', and that the admission of women was 'productive of nothing but good to the institution'.[31] Clearly, women were gradually becoming accepted in some quarters within the medical schools. This professional support was essential for women who were new to the male-dominated medical fields. On graduation in June 1899, Lynn won the prestigious Hudson Prize for the Adelaide student who was awarded the highest marks in the final medical examination, as well as the silver medal.

Senia Paseta has suggested that 'education signified more than intellectual capital'. The advantages of an extended education were manifold. Through educational opportunities a vocal and energetic generation of men and women came to the forefront of national life.[32] Because Lynn was educated with Catholic men and women, she may have imbibed some of the intoxicating mix of nationalism and *fin de siècle* enthusiasm for the future. Ireland in the 1890s was in the midst of a cultural and political revival and the university environment was a political one, where new ideas were exchanged. Sometimes nationalism and suffragism became intertwined. One commentator suggested that higher education would allow women to lead a 'richer, freer life and made fuller personal development possible, freeing women from mere eccentricity, political faddism, philanthropic hysteria and busy-body shallow restlessness.'[33] It can be argued that Lynn's university experience prepared her and some of her contemporaries for the turmoil of the 1910s. For some, their university careers propelled them into political activity and philanthropic professions.

While Lynn is probably the most well known of the pre-1900 female medical graduates, between 1891 and 1900 twenty-five women were awarded a medical degree from the RUI and six received their Masters in medicine.[34] In 1898–99, there were five female students at Cecilia Street, and this tripled to fifteen by 1900–1901. In 1899 Winifred Dickson, who had become the first woman Fellow of the Royal College of Surgeons in Ireland in 1893, suggested in the *Alexandra College Magazine* that female doctors brought practical merits to the profession.[35] The reputation of Ireland in providing opportunities for medical women was further enhanced when Dickson became an examiner in Midwifery and Gynaecology at the Royal College of Surgeons in Ireland in 1896.

The *Englishwoman's Review* reported that 'Ireland has again led the way in the medical progress of women'.[36] While Ireland had a remarkable reputation in the medical education of women, it was still difficult for them to obtain employment.

EARLY PROFESSIONAL EXPERIENCES

In 1902, just after Lynn had qualified from the Catholic University, an ode by Mac Aodh challenged the readers of *St Stephen's*, the university's student magazine, to 'vindicate the Lady-Medico.'[37]

> *Ode to the Lady Medicals*
> Though all the world's a stage and we are acting
> Yet still I think your part is not dissecting.
> To me the art of making apple tarts
> Would suit you better than those 'horrid parts'.
> ... And as for learning chemistry and that,
> 'Twould be a nicer thing to trim a hat.
> I know your aims are true,
> But tell me is there any *need* of you?

Qualifying was only the first step towards becoming a professional. It was necessary to obtain employment in one's chosen profession. In an oversupplied profession like medicine, this was often a difficult task. Frequently, women 'lacked the needed medical connections'.[38] Lynn was refused a position as a resident doctor in the prestigious Adelaide Hospital, which was under Protestant management. The other doctors objected to a female colleague, even though she had been elected as a resident doctor. It was not until May 1913 that the medical board allowed female students to apply for residence at the hospital.[39] Despite difficulties with the Adelaide, Lynn gained valuable experience in the Rotunda, the Royal Victoria Eye and Ear, and Sir Patrick Dun's between 1906 and 1916. After postgraduate study in the United States, Lynn was to become the third female, in 1909, to be awarded the fellowship of the Royal College of Surgeons. This should have ensured a high medical standing when hospital positions were limited.

Lynn's early career is many ways resembles those of some of the early female academics. In her biography of Eileen Power, a well-known historian who was a contemporary of Lynn, Maxine Berg described these early professional women as 'Victorian in dress and hairstyle, feminist and committed to the campaign for women's suffrage, and single-mindedly academic'.[40] Lynn had both the leisure time and financial wherewithal to devote herself to many causes. She was also somewhat old fashioned, with her disapproval of trousers and make-up. Her professional ambition is suggested by her pursuit of extra qualifications as well as international experience. This cosmopolitan approach was also evident in the 1920s when she visited various paediatric institutions in the United States.

Between 1910 and 1916, she was a clinical assistant in the Royal Victoria Eye and Ear Hospital, but was not allowed to return after the 1916 Rising. Another female doctor, Dr Georgina Prosser, was appointed to replace her.[41] Lynn's work there ensured that she developed a reputation as an eye specialist or ophthalmologist. This was to be particularly useful in her general practice at Rathmines.

RATHMINES

Lynn was to spend her career in the comfortable, middle-class environment of 9 Belgrave Road, Rathmines, in the south side of the city of Dublin. The Plunkett family, who were to become heavily involved in nationalist movements in the 1910s, had built much of this area in the post-Famine period. Lynn came to Rathmines in 1902–03, and remained there until the year of her death. In the early twentieth century, it was a mixed township, since 60 per cent of its residents were members of various Protestant churches.[42] Like many professional women, she lived in rented accommodation. She shared her house with a boarder, Frances Margaret Cooke, a member of the Church of Ireland from Waterford aged 44. Like most people of her class, she also had a servant; Bridget Cuffe, a Roman Catholic, from Ferns, County Wexford.[43] As a professional woman in an all-female household she would have enjoyed privileges and luxuries which were denied to many.

At the beginning of the twentieth century, Dublin had the fifth highest mortality rate in the world; clearly there was great need for medical expertise as well as improvements in living conditions.[44] The appalling death rate was a reflection on the pervasive poverty of the city. Lynn's professional career was to be devoted to the health and welfare of the poor of Dublin.

CONCLUSION

Writing in 1902, the maverick politician Frank Hugh O'Donnell proclaimed that female students were 'fit for nothing under heaven except casting flowers before the Banner of the Sodality. If they were even brought up to be skilled teachers, zenana doctors [they would only care for females], etc., they might be able to be of some use proportionate to their silent and pitiable self-sacrifice'.[45]

More realistically, Anne Jellicoe, one of the founders of Alexandra College, wanted to give Irish women an education which 'would fit them to adorn an exalted position or enable them under adverse circumstances to enter on a career of usefulness and independence'.[46] After an extensive and expensive education, Lynn was fit and ready for a life filled with independence and usefulness. This ophthalmologist would receive the full glare of public scrutiny during the 1910s. The consciousness-raising potential of her lengthy education was evident in her professional career. Lynn's socio-economic advantages provided her with the opportunity to establish a medical practice. However, nothing could have prepared her for the events of that decade.

NOTES

1 Details on Robert Lynn's career are based on Representative Church Body Library RCBL MS 61/2/15.
2 T. P. O'Neill, 'From famine to near famine' in *Studia Hibernica*, vol. 1, 1961, pp. 161–71.
3 LD, 28 April 1937.
4 Donald E. Jordan, *Land and Popular Politics in Ireland: County Mayo from the Plantation to the Land War* (Cambridge, 1994), p. 295.

5 Janet Te Brake, 'Irish peasant women in revolt: the Land League years' in *Irish Historical Studies*, May 1992, vol. xxvii, no. 109, pp. 63–80, p. 66.
6 See Chapter 3 for Lynn's involvement in political philanthropy in the 1910s and 1920s.
7 Adrian Wilson, 'Conflict, consensus and charity: politics and the provincial voluntary hospitals in the eighteenth century' in *English Historical Review*, June 1996, pp. 599–619, p. 618.
8 LD, 14 Sept., 1944.
9 *The Medical Register 1881* (London, 1881), p. 748. Dr Smartt had received his licentiate from the Royal College of Surgeons in 1855 and was awarded the Licentiate in Midwifery from the King's and Queen's College of Physicians in Ireland in 1860. The following year he was awarded an MD (Masters degree in Medicine) from the University of St Andrews. Hence, he was well qualified to practise medicine. Medb Ruane, 'Kathleen Lynn (1874–1955)', in Mary Cullen and Maria Luddy (eds), *Female Activists. Irish Women and Change, 1900–1960* (Dublin, 2001), pp. 61–88, p. 62.
10 Lyons, Brief Lives p. 159.
11 Ruane, 'Lynn', p. 62.
12 E. Jordan, *Land and Popular Politics in Ireland* pp. 295–96.
13 'Spent aft tearing up old letters, kept those of when "Prince of Wales" was in Cong. Mother's are so motherly.' LD, 2 Sept. 1944; Ruane, 'Lynn' p. 63.
14 LD, 1 Feb. 1936.
15 See Anne V. O'Connor, and Susan M. Parkes, *Gladly Learn and Gladly Teach: A History of Alexandra College and School, Dublin 1866–1966* (Dublin, 1983).
16 Linda Clark, *Schooling the Daughters of Marianne* (New York, 1984), p. 16.
17 Kathleen Lynch, 'The universal and particular: gender, class and reproduction in second-level Schools', in *UCD Women's Studies Forum Working Paper*, no. 3, 1987, p. 7.
18 Ruane, 'Lynn', p. 65.
19 Mary E. Daly, 'Women in the Irish Free State, 1922–39: the interaction between politics and ideology', in Joan Hoff and Maureen Coulter (eds), *Irish Women's Voices. Past and Present. Journal of Women's History*, vol. 6, no. 4/vol. 7, no. 1 (winter/spring), (Indiana, 1995), pp. 99–116, pp. 106–7.
20 Barbara Miller Solomon, *In the Company of Educated Women: A History of Women and Higher Education in America* (New Haven, 1985), p. 70.
21 Thomas J. Morrissey, *Towards a National University: William Delany SJ (1835–1924). An Era of Initiative in Irish Education* (Dublin, 1983), pp. 279–87.
22 Royal College of Science Registers B65 in UCD Archives; RUI Calendar 1890–1899.
23 In 1885 Dr Jex-Blake established the Edinburgh Hospital and Dispensary for Women and Children, where most of the staff were female, just like St Ultan's. For Jex-Blake's career see *British Medical Journal*, 20 Jan. 1912, pp. 165–66, and *Medical Press*, 12 Jan. 1912, Kirkpatrick Biographical Archive, Royal College of Physicians; Sophia Jex-Blake MD, *Medical Women: A Thesis and A History* (Second Edition, Edinburgh and London, 1886). The

Royal College of Physicians copy of Jex-Blake's book contains the following inscription: 'compliments of the Executive Committee of the National Association for Promoting the Medical Education of Women.' Jex-Blake was awarded her licentiate from the Royal College of Physicians in Ireland in 1877. Shirley Roberts has written a modern biography, see *Sophia Jex-Blake: A Woman Pioneer in Nineteenth-Century Medical Reform* (London, New York, 1993).

24 Sophia Jex-Blake, 'Medicine as a Profession for Women', in Susan Groag Bell and Karen Offen (eds), *Women, the Family and Freedom: The Debate in the Documents* (Stanford, 1983) p. 477.
25 David Mitchell, *A 'Peculiar' Place: The Adelaide Hospital, Dublin: Its Time, Places and Personalities, 1839–1989* (Dublin, 1989), p. 258.
26 Ruane, 'Lynn', p. 66.
27 Mitchell, *Adelaide*, p. 258.
28 Ruane, 'Lynn', p. 67.
29 F.O.C. Meenan, *Cecilia Street: The Catholic University School of Medicine, 1855–1931* (Dublin, 1987), p. 82.
30 Medical Directory, 1910.
31 Robertson Commission 1902, Appendix to 3rd Report, vol. xxxii, cd. 1229, p. 333.
32 Senia Paseta, *Before the Revolution: Nationalism, Social Change and Ireland's Catholic Elite, 1879–1922* (Cork, 1999), p. 6.
33 Cited in Eibhlín Breathnach, 'A History of the Movement for Higher Education in Dublin, 1860–1912' (MA, UCD, 1981), p. 146.
34 Robertson Commission 1902, pp. 282–83.
35 *Alexandra College Magazine*, June 1899, pp. 368–75.
36 Irene Finn, 'Women in the medical profession in Ireland, 1876–1919', in Bernadette Whelan (ed.), *Women and Paid Work in Ireland, 1500–1930* (Dublin, 2000), pp. 102–19, p. 110.
37 *St Stephen's*, March 1902, p. 93.
38 Regina Markell Morantz-Sanchez, *Sympathy and Science: Women Physicians in American Medicine* (Oxford, 1985), p. 145.
39 Mitchell, *Adelaide*, p. 148.
40 Maxine Berg, 'Foreword: Eileen Power, 1889–1940', in Eileen Power, *Medieval Women* (Cambridge, 1995), pp. ix–xxvi, p. xi.
41 Gearóid Crookes, *Dublin's Eye and Ear: The Making of a Monument* (Dublin, 1993), pp. 105 and 88.
42 R.B. McDowell, *Crisis and Decline: Southern Unionists in Ireland* (Dublin, 2000), pp. 4–5.
43 1911 Census, Dublin 60/26, National Archives of Ireland (NAI).
44 Mary E. Daly, *Dublin, the Deposed Capital* (Cork, 1984), pp. 240–76.
45 Frank Hugh O'Donnell, *The Ruin of Education in Ireland* (London, 1902), pp. 151–53.
46 *Alexandra College Magazine*, Dec. 1918, p. 38.

CHAPTER TWO

Rebellious womanhood 1912–30[1]

THE 1910S WERE A decade of growing politicisation for Lynn. Through the suffrage movement as well as James Larkin's Irish Transport and General Workers' Union (ITGWU) and the socialism advocated by James Connolly, Lynn was to be politicised and energised. On 21 August 1911, the Irish Women's Suffrage Federation was formed. It was the suffrage movement which provided Lynn with her first taste of politics.

The atmosphere of the 1910s provided the crucible for Lynn's political education. By 1912, she was 38 years old and quite well established professionally. Within a decade she was at the forefront of a national movement which sought Irish independence. For Lynn suffragism, socialism and medicine were intertwined. Medico-political activities, such as teaching first aid to Cumann na mBan, the women's wing of the nationalistic Irish Volunteers, provided Lynn with a much-appreciated role. She was based in City Hall during the 1916 Rising, in full view of Dublin Castle, the centre of British power in Ireland; her role as chief medical officer, as well as her subsequent imprisonment, needs to be carefully dissected. The eventual outbreak of the flu pandemic in 1918 gave her the opportunity to utilise her medical skills in the face of an increasingly tense political situation.

SUFFRAGISM AND NATIONALISM

Politically, Lynn moved from suffragism to socialism and then to republicanism. The suffrage movement in Ireland, like suffrage movements elsewhere, attracted educated, middle-class men and women like Lynn. Some of the suffragists, like Lynn, had endured professional discrimination. Lynn was all too aware of the

Rebellious womanhood, 1912–30

politics of exclusion. Despite the small numbers of activists, these suffragists were to exert a significant influence on Irish politics. Lynn was a member of the executive committee of the Irish Women's Suffrage and Local Government Association (IWSLGA) from 1903, and remained on the executive until 1916.[2]

Furthermore, increasing interest in public health and the possibilities for improvement interested Lynn both professionally and personally. Women's traditional role as carers had facilitated their entry to the medical profession, but they still did not have formal political power. As educated women, it is not surprising that most medical women were in favour of suffrage. In 1908, 538 medical women in the United Kingdom of Great Britain and Ireland were in favour of extending the franchise to women, while 15 were against.[3] Lynn was a member of the radical British Women's Social and Political Union (WSPU) from 1908 and it is clear that she was on friendly terms with the suffragist Sylvia Pankhurst.[4] The WSPU was an 'explicitly militant organisation', and in 1908 IWSLGA members took part in a large suffrage demonstration in London.[5] In June 1912 a mass meeting was held in Dublin in order to demand that female suffrage be included in the Home Rule bill of that year. Lynn shared a platform with other women who were to become prominent in various women's causes, such as Jennie Wyse Power, then vice president of Sinn Féin, and Delia Larkin of the Irish Women's Workers' Union.[6] In later years, Lynn admitted that she had become interested in the Women's Suffrage Movement through 'Mr. and Mrs. Haslam and quite sympathised with the militant side of it.'[7]

Anna and Thomas Haslam[8] were the personification of activism having been involved in virtually every feminist campaign from the 1860s. Of Quaker upbringing, they typified the kind of people suffrage attracted with their concern for equality and their middle-class background. Lynn knew the Haslams through the Irish Women's Suffrage and Local Government Association, which included fellow female physicians Katherine Maguire and Elizabeth Tennant. Furthermore, Lynn's professional skills forged further links with prominent suffragists. In December 1913 the *Irish Citizen* reported that Hanna Sheehy Skeffington was 'under the care of Dr Kathleen Lynn'. Lynn's report, read at the Irish Women's

Franchise League, stated that Mrs Skeffington's heart showed 'signs of improvement' and that her 'sleeplessness' which concerned them, was abating.[9]

It was through her professional work that Lynn was to meet those most associated with nationalism. While doing locum work for Dr Katherine Maguire, Lynn was called to Surrey House, Constance Markievicz's home in 1913. Helena Molony, Markievicz's friend, was ill.[10] Lynn was attracted to political organisations through Molony's magnetism. She stayed with Lynn in Rathmines and they 'used to have long talks' which 'converted' Lynn to the 'National movement.' Lynn described Molony as 'a very clever and attractive girl with a tremendous power of making friends.'[11]

Molony was an actress at the Abbey Theatre and, more significantly in this context, a very active trade unionist; she assisted strikers during the 1913 Lockout of workers. As co-founder and editor of *Bean na hÉireann* she espoused republican and suffragist ideals. Furthermore, Molony was active in Inghínídhe na hÉireann and Cumann na mBan.[12] Inghínídhe na hÉireann had been established by Maud Gonne in 1900 and consisted primarily of nationalist women. Cumann na mBan was established in 1914 as an auxiliary group for the Irish Volunteers. Most of the ninety women who fought during Easter Week were Cumann na mBan members, but about thirty were part of the more radical Irish Citizen Army.[13]

Many years after the 1916 Rising, Lynn commented: 'I was converted to republicanism through suffrage. I saw that people got the wrong impression about suffrage and that led me to examine the Irish question.'[14] Hence, one form of injustice led her to examine another. Nationalists argued that Ireland's political connection with Britain was a form of injustice and that Ireland did not benefit from its connection to one of the most developed countries in the world. Nationalistic socialists believed that Ireland was penalised economically by the British connection.

The Irish Citizen Army (ICA) or 'workers' militia'[15] had been formed in 1913 in order to protect striking workers. This citizen militia was, W.K. Anderson suggests, akin to Sylvia Pankhurst's 'People's Army', which was founded in the same year.[16] This linking of suffrage and labour was to prove a potent mix during

1916. Lynn was affected by the equality of treatment that characterised the Irish Citizen Army. It is entirely appropriate that the gender-neutral term 'citizen' was used since this suggested that there was no differentiation between men and women. James Connolly was known for his support of suffrage, unlike many of his co-revolutionaries. He linked 'sex-consciousness' to a 'deep feeling of social consciousness' and 'civic consciousness'. Connolly believed that awareness of sexual inequality made people aware of other inequalities in society. Furthermore, he suggested that the 'more intellectual women broke out into revolt'.[19] It was the better educated women who were aware of civic disabilities, and the ICA boasted several middle-class women such as Lynn and Madeleine ffrench-Mullen. This awareness of social and political wants affected Lynn. Many years later she admitted that she 'knew and admired James Connolly'.[17] Lynn was asked by Connolly to teach first aid to the ICA. She went on to become a captain and chief medical officer in the organisation.

Both Lynn and her relative and 'great friend' Markievicz worked in the soup kitchens during the 1913 Lockout. Working in the soup kitchens would bring Lynn into close contact with the families of unemployed or poorly paid workers in Dublin whose plight was later exposed by the playwright Sean O'Casey. These charitable activities, or 'political philanthropy', were to push Lynn further along the road to revolution. Probably the most famous of the 1916 women was Markievicz. Lynn thought 'Markievicz was a grand soul. She was brimming with enthusiasm and was not like other people. Although you might gather from her manner that she was fantastic, she was full of sound sense and was quite practical.'[18]

When the artist and nationalist Susan Mitchell saw ffrench-Mullen speak at a political meeting, Mitchell's friend Johnny thought ffrench-Mullen 'was a man. She would be proud.'[20] With her closely-cropped hair, ffrench-Mullen looked boyish. Lynn was clearly very feminine with her long hair, frequently tied up in plaits. The relationship between Lynn and ffrench-Mullen was intimate as they shared many interests. Was it a sexual relationship? Despite Lynn's willingness to discuss many private matters in her diary, there is no indication that the relationship between the two friends was sexual. The links between women with similar outlooks, albeit different denominational backgrounds (ffrench-Mullen was a Roman Catholic), should not surprise us given that these women shared an interest in children. Furthermore, they were both committed nationalists. The close cooperation, on a personal level, between Lynn and ffrench-Mullen, was replicated on a national level.

Suffragism and nationalism were frequently intertwined. The Irish Citizen made the connections between the two clear. It reported that the Irish Women's Reform League (IWRL) was very antagonistic to the force-feeding 'of suffrage and political prisoners'. During the political turmoil of the late 1910s, Lynn was to object to the force-feeding of nationalists such as Thomas Ashe. In 1913, the Irish Women's Reform League collected 188 signatories, including those of medical practitioners Lynn, Katherine Maguire, Ella Webb, Alice Barry and Mary Strangman, to protest against force-feeding.[21] Particularly criticised was the Prisoners (Temporary Discharge for Ill Health) Act of 1913, known as the Cat and Mouse Act because of the constant re-capturing of released prisoners by the authorities. Lynn cited the case of Gladys Evans, a British woman, who was re-imprisoned six times.[22] Evans was exhausted when released, and Lynn described the imprisonment experience as 'appalling'. She suggested to fellow suffragette Hanna Sheehy Skeffington that 'Irishmen & women see to it that there shall be no repetition of such barbarism'.[23]

However, there were divisions over the correct tactics and Lynn was caught up in the confused political crises on the eve of the First World War. A correspondent of Hanna Sheehy Skeffington, and fellow suffragette, Marguerite Palmer, suggested that Lynn was 'spending her substance on bags of flour' and had not 'come up to scratch yet.' Palmer wanted Lynn to speak at 'open-air meetings' of the Irish Women's Reform League, but she had other commitments. Lynn, Palmer suggested, was 'splendid on suffrage – strong on W.S.P.U. [Women's Social and Progressive Union] declaring *no* truce during the war, which is refreshing.' It was hoped that Lynn would join the league since her 'Nationalist and Labourite' tendencies made her an unlikely supporter of British organisations. Finally, Palmer declared that Lynn had 'good stuff in her undoubtedly, but is unwary.'[24] One of the biggest difficulties facing suffrage organisations on the eve of the war was whether there should be a truce on suffrage matters for the duration of the war. Clearly Lynn believed that suffrage should not be pursued regardless of international turmoil. Like many nationalists she thought that an independent Irish state would confer equal rights on all.

Lynn's connections with suffrage, nationalist and labour activists such as Connolly, Molony and Sheehy Skeffington politicised her. A photograph of the National Aid Women in the Kilmainham Gaol archives shows Lynn and ffrench-Mullen at the front.[25]

THE 1916 RISING

The role and importance of Lynn during the Easter Rising were the result of her prominence in the ICA prior to 1916. On St Patrick's Day, 17 March 1916, a month before the Rising, Lynn saw a 'Volunteer Parade in [the] street and heard bands'. She enthusiastically declared, 'Thank God Ireland is alive & throbbing.'[26] 'The Rising was led by those who had been beyond the interest or appeal of the parliamentarians – Fenians, socialists, Gaelic Leaguers, GAA members, politicized women, the young', according to Alvin Jackson.[27]

About two weeks before the insurrection, Connolly asked Lynn to take him out to the coast, 'along the Howth Road but not as far as Howth. He wanted to do some reconnoitring. He was looking out to find some suitable place for the Germans to land or to have an encampment. On another occasion I drove about three men of the Citizen Army to a place in Sutton [north Dublin] where there were British rifles.' Closer to the date even more preparations were afoot. 'One night in Holy Week I went out with the car to St Enda's [the all-Irish school established by Pearse] and there they loaded it up with ammunition and put some theatrical stuff on top of it, hoping to get through. Willie Pearse [Pádraig's brother] and I brought it in and landed it safely in Liberty Hall where there were many willing hands to unload it.' Lynn's home in Belgrave Road was used to store ammunition from Belfast.

Lynn was very open about her involvement in the Rising. Clearly, her help was appreciated.

> On Holy Thursday, Connolly and the Citizen Army made me a present as a token of gratitude for the help I had given in connection with medical preparations for the Rising, providing first aid equipment, medical dressings and so on. It was a gold brooch in the form of a fibula [leg bone] and it is still my most treasured possession. The inscription is as follows: "To Dr Kathleen Lynn from the men and women of the I.C.A.". . . the Cumann na mBan for the same reason presented me with a pair of silver candlesticks and an ink bottle, similarly inscribed.[28]

Lynn was to treasure these gifts. Her hidden work was frequently forgotten about once the Rising was over.

Despite her activity, Lynn was not fully aware of the precise plans for the Rising as they were not openly discussed. She did not know until two days before the insurrection where she was going to be stationed, but this was to be expected given the air of secrecy and uncertainty. On Sunday, 23 April, Easter Sunday, in Liberty Hall, she spotted all of the leaders 'coming and going', while 'Connolly was a bit worried and uncertain how things were going to turn out.' Nonetheless, 'he and the Citizen Army were determined to go out and fight'.[29]

A decade after the Rising, Markievicz recalled that she went off with Lynn in Lynn's car:

> We carried a large store of first aid necessities and drove off through the quiet, dusty streets and across the river, reaching City Hall just at the very moment Commandant Séan Connolly and his little troop of men and women swung round the corner and raised his gun and shot the policeman who barred the way . . . I did not meet Dr Lynn again till my release, when her car met me, and she welcomed me to her house where she cared [for] me and fed me up and looked after me till I had recovered from the evil effects of the English prison system.[30]

Markievicz served on Stephen's Green with ffrench-Mullen who was in charge of the Red Cross. Like Lynn, ffrench-Mullen took care of the sick and prisoners.[31]

Significantly, the ICA permitted women to bear arms, then considered very radical. In effect, they were fighting soldiers. Lynn was assigned to City Hall with the position of captain, while ffrench-Mullen was a lieutenant. At City Hall, where the actor and trade unionist, Sean Connolly, was in command, Lynn and his girlfriend, Helena Molony, received their first taste of the tragedy that rebellions bring. Lynn described the event.

> It was a beautiful day, the sun was hot and we were not long there when we noticed Sean Connolly coming towards us, walking upright, although we had been advised to crouch and take cover as much as possible. We suddenly saw him fall mortally wounded by a sniper's bullet from the Castle. First aid was useless. He died almost immediately.

In the 1950s, Nora Connolly O'Brien, James Connolly's daughter, spoke about Lynn's activities during 1916. Connolly thought that Lynn was the 'most amazing' of all the ICA women. He suggested that with 'her early training and environment', it was remarkable that she 'should find her niche in the Citizen Army, be so thoroughly at home with them and be so completely accepted by them [. . . it was] something to be constantly amazed at.' Furthermore

> The members of the Citizen Army, who were perhaps more famed for the toughness of their qualities than for the delicacy of their perceptions, were swift to recognise this calm serenity of Dr Lynn, and won comfort and assurance from it many times . . . Those who were there with her remember and often tell of her calmness and serenity while on the roof of the City Hall with bullets smacking all round her she straightened and covered the body of Sean Connolly.

Lynn's 'quiet yet authoritative manner' as well as her 'serene faith' were to enable her to endure the trauma of the Rising.[32] There is a class element in these comments. Lynn's involvement in a socialist republican movement is seen as surprising, yet her medical experience, as well as her personality, facilitated her accession to a leadership position in the ICA. This begs the question, how socialist was the ICA? Clearly, the old assumptions about class surface in the comments of Nora Connolly O'Brien, the daughter of

Ireland's most famous and most international socialist. Lynn's 'serenity' and her ability to 'comfort' others possibly derived from her professional experience. Even at this stage we see Lynn taking charge, and this authority was all the more evident in her political and medical career.

Lynn thought that Sean Connolly's death had a 'demoralising effect on the City Hall men'. When they were eventually captured after spending the night at the garrison, Lynn told the British officer that she was a doctor. He thought she was there only in a medical capacity. When she informed him that she was a member of the Citizen Army it 'surprised him very much'.[33] The occupants of City Hall were marched to Ship St Barracks.

The real impact of the Rising was its aftermath. Once the Rising had been quelled, activists endured weeks or months of prison in close proximity. This experience helped to politicise those who may have been lukewarm in their commitment. Furthermore, the imprisonment of many and the executions of the leaders affected the population at large. Michael Laffan suggests that the aftermath of the Rising 'saw a process of wholesale conversion, along with a pattern of retrospective endorsement of the defeated rebels and of their objectives.'[34]

AFTERMATH OF THE RISING

Immediately after capture, Lynn was in Ship Street Barracks beside Dublin Castle for nearly a week. They had a 'good dinner' the first day but 'after that, the food got slacker and slacker' until they were forced to subsist on 'ship's biscuits and water'. Despite the grim conditions, Lynn noted any small act of kindness and she described the old military sergeant as a 'kind old boy'. He gave them oranges which were greatly appreciated. However, the toilet facilities left a lot to be desired. She described the lavatory accommodation as 'appalling' and their blankets were 'crawling with lice'. When they objected to lavatory accommodation they were told 'it was good enough for us, that lice, fleas & typhoid should content us.'[35] Betraying her comfortable background as well as her medical concerns, Lynn admitted she was 'very sensitive to that sort of thing'.

Her co-prisoners, on the other hand, were less concerned. 'I used to marvel how the others girls seemed to sleep. They did not seem to mind.'[36] Furthermore, Lynn's desire to maintain good physical health is clear:

> Asked M.O. for baths & exercise. Saw men, prisoners with him, [Halpin, a rebel, who was 'brought in, utterly exhausted having been in chimney, without food'] who were much worse off than we, about 30 in a small lock up room, with absolutely nothing in it but a wooden platform, no bedding, no washing apparatus – herded like a lot of swine, poor fellows, M.O. promised baths & exercise & was really kind.[37]

From this diary entry it is clear that Lynn was both compassionate and pragmatic. She saw that hygiene was essential and that exercise was important both physically and psychologically. Furthermore, her diaries were therapeutic for someone who was used to a comfortable environment. Her requests clearly indicate her concern for others, and she noticed that the male prisoners were worse off. In general, few females were imprisoned – a total of ninety – and even fewer (six) were deported. Lynn, Markievicz, Molony, Marie Perolz, Kathleen Clarke and Brigid Foley all spent time in Britain because of their heavy involvement in 1916.[38]

Kathleen Clarke, the wife of Tom Clarke, one of the signatories of the 1916 Proclamation, has written a memoir of her republican activities. After the execution of the leaders of the Rising, Clarke 'formed the first committee of the Irish Republican Prisoners Dependants' Fund'.[39] Lynn was heavily involved in its various activities and was particularly critical of the ill treatment meted out to prisoners and the consequent suffering borne by their family and friends.

On 1 May Lynn was taken to Kilmainham, where most of the prisoners were being held. This was an indication of her high ranking position in the Rising. Kilmainham was used to detain the leaders of the Rising. In the afternoon, fifty men and twelve women were taken to Richmond Barracks. Not surprisingly, given her anti-British and republican outlook, Lynn noted abuses committed by the British Army. 'In [Dublin] Castle officer told soldier to prod Nurse Treston with bayonet for not at once falling into line saying he had seen her shoot 6 police.'[40] The men stayed at Richmond Barracks, while the women were transferred to Kilmainham. Kathleen Clarke painted a grim picture of Kilmainham. It 'presented a scene of gloom and decay. It had been abandoned as a prison for many years. A damp smell pervaded the whole place, and the only light was candles in jamjars.'[41]

While Lynn and the other republican women like Sighle Humphreys were being transferred to Kilmainham, there was a 'great ovation', 'only the separation women hooted'.[42] These women were dependent on the separation allowance provided by the British government while their relations fought in the First World War. Lynn, ffrench-Mullen and Molony shared a tiny cell. It was 'such joy, cheerfully we do with one basin of water for washings, hog wash of cocoa & dog biscuits for b.fast. Madam Markiev. here in solitary. We had a loan of her comb & soap.' Lynn commented that there were about seventy women in Kilmainham, mainly ICA and Cumann na mBan.[43] The following day, 3 May, the shooting of the leaders began. She wrote simply: 'We hear they have shot members of the Provisional Govt.'[44] Despite the grim conditions, and in a piece of pathetic fallacy, Lynn delighted in the fact that 'ever since Republic proclaimed weather has been glorious'. Lynn maintained her calm authority while in Kilmainham. She was assertive in demanding immediate release for fellow prisoners. On 6 May, after nearly a week in jail she noted,

> M & I asked to see governor, spoke to him abt. Ch. to-morrow, begged him to have young girls examined immediately & released – so far none have been examined for 3 days.[45]

Lynn did not want young women detained in Kilmainham, hence her desire that they be released at once. But how did Lynn survive the trauma of imprisonment? It is clear from her diaries that her devout faith sustained her. A Church of Ireland clergyman refused to have a service at Kilmainham as 'there was no place'. Lynn 'insisted & he had it, a very hurried affair, over in 10 min'. She also asked for a prayer book, which she never received.[46] Lynn was allowed to have matins on Sunday and a celebration of service at her request. However, ffrench-Mullen was not allowed to attend mass because she had not made an official statement regarding her involvement in 1916 to the authorities. The closeness between Lynn and ffrench-Mullen was very evident during their sojourn in Kilmainham. While Lynn was at service, 'M was getting very lonely'.[47]

The effect of being in Kilmainham when prisoners were being executed 'was a harrowing experience', Lynn admitted. She could hear the shootings in the morning and Markievicz, who had been condemned, was in the cell above them. It is clear that she saw the rebels as martyrs for a cause. Here Lynn's Christianity merged with nationalism. 'Later saw Fr. Albert [a Franciscan]. He was with Mallin, Heuston & Colbert this mg. They were wonderful in their consciousness of the Unseen & went to deaths with prayers on lips. He could have wished to be in their place. We were so sad after he left. We looked out on the hills and thought of psalms wh. have been such a comfort to us.'[48] The following day, when her family advised her to give up her republican friends, she said she would follow her conscience. That evening Lynn heard pitiful crying; 'it was Miss Gifford, [Sidney, sister of Grace the newly-wed wife of the executed leader, Joseph Plunkett][49] her brother told her that 2 brothers in law were shot, Macdonagh & Plunkett. Kind matron let me go to her for a little. Just at bedtime we were scurried off in Black Maria to Mtjoy, [Mountjoy Prison] travelled with Countess Plunkett. Went by bye streets for fear of a rescue.'[50] Given the continuous threat of hearing shots and news about executions, it was probably a relief for Lynn to be out of Kilmainham. Her diaries portray the fear which pervaded the institution. However, she was to spend nearly six weeks in Mountjoy. Her first diary entry from Mountjoy is revealing. 'Mtjoy clean and comfortable, but I'd give £10,000 for Kilmainham & Madelene. Matrons v. kind.'[51] Charitably Lynn praised those who guarded them. Despite the relative comforts of Mountjoy, she would prefer to be in grim Kilmainham with her beloved Madeleine.

> We were hailed rather with joy by the wardresses because we were interesting prisoners. We were not like ordinary prisoners.

I got quite fond of the wardress who looked after me. She was quite kindly. We discovered that, when the suffragettes were there, they had made little holes in the plaster under the pipes so that, if one lay down on the floor, one could talk to the person in the next cell.

While in Kilmainham, Countess Plunkett was next door to Lynn and distraught because her son, Joseph, had been executed. They spoke to each other during the night and this seemed to help the Countess. In time, the prison regime relaxed and prisoners were allowed to receive presents. True to form, all Lynn desired was 'clean bread and butter'. Lynn spent six weeks in Mountjoy, lost a lot of weight and was less than 110 pounds; normally she was 124 pounds (fifty-six kilograms). For someone of five foot seven inches, the weight loss made her look frail, though she was sturdy. Lynn maintained that she was 'not upset' by what she experienced.

Throughout her diaries, she refers to various political events; the shooting of prisoners, the attitude of the British state and the response of the detainees. If anything, like others involved in the Rising, her experiences in the spring and early summer of 1916 deepened her desire to do something about the political connection between Britain and Ireland. Because Lynn kept notes while in prison, which she later transferred to her diary, we can gauge her moods and aspirations. For example, while being held at Ship Street Barracks, near Dublin Castle, a 'terribly excited prostitute [was] brought in, nearly mad, her brother shot Tues. & she had gone to see body. We couldn't quiet her. Two soldiers came in, one held revolver to her head, other twisted her wrists, Emer [Molony] jumped up, told him to stop & had revolver turned on her. They were brutal. D.G. they left. I gave poor soul morphia hypo. She lay down & slept beside me.'[52] Lynn's compassion and professional skills were essential but she could do little about the response of the British state to the Rising. By May, when the leaders of the Rising were being executed, she asked, 'What other country shoots its prisoners in cold blood!'[53] The impact of her prison experiences would be felt long after 1916.

The rebellion became an international news item as some American journalists visited the prisoners in Mountjoy.[54] Lynn remembered 'a lady among them who asked us were we "diehards". At that time I did not know what diehards meant. She said afterwards that she never came across such a stupid set as we were. I think our brains were comatose after what we had been through and they refused to work for us. We were not at all up to the mark and as snappy as they would have liked us to be. They got the impression that we were a poor lot.' Fortunately, not everybody shared this view. Later, American aid would prove to be very useful for those pursuing Irish independence, as nationalists went to the US in the time-honoured republican tradition. Lynn would use American links to fund St Ultan's Hospital for Infants.

While American journalists may have thought that the rebels were 'stupid', Lynn's family was horrified at her activities. Her uncomprehending father and sister visited Mountjoy.

> A very black Friday. Fardie & Nan were here, oh, so reproachful, they wouldn't listen to me & looked as if they would cast me off forever. How sorry I am for their sorrow! Erin needs very big sacrifices. I am glad they go home to-morrow. Why do they always misunderstand me?[55]

Their dismay was entirely predictable given the radicalism of her activity. Daughters of Church of Ireland clergymen were not usually incarcerated in Mountjoy. Her loyalist friends were particularly concerned about her. They managed to convince the authorities that she was insane and not a political figure. It would have been easier to accept that she was suffering from temporary insanity, than to admit that she was a prominent political figure. The *Freeman's Journal* published a letter from 'a loyalist and unionist' which claimed that Lynn was involved in the Rising as a doctor only. The writer praised Lynn's work at the Royal Victoria Eye and Ear where she gave her services free three times a week. Furthermore, Lynn was described as 'an honourable Christian lady'. Hagiographically, the writer suggested that the 'present generation has seen few equals of Dr Kathleen Lynn and no superiors'. She was known 'lovingly' as the doctor.[56] Lynn's reaction to the letter is unknown. The writer may have been a former colleague at the Royal Victoria Eye and Ear Hospital. It must have been mortifying for Lynn's family to have her connected with the militant events of 1916. Nonetheless, all was not grim for Lynn in Mountjoy. On 17 May she wrote, there 'hasn't been much to note, nothing happens here, but everyone is kind (not governor etc.) & we have many gifts of fruit, flowers etc. fr. kind friends'.[57]

Despite all the protestations of her friends, Lynn was deported and sent to Coltsford, near Bath, in the west of England. Jennie Wyse Power, who went on to become a senator in the Irish Free State, arranged for Lynn to work in England with an Irish doctor named Brian Cusack.[58] He was a friend of Wyse Power and it was hoped that Lynn would be out of trouble there. As Cusack recounted, many years later, Lynn announced, the second morning after her arrival in Bath, that she had to go and see ffrench-Mullen in London. He discovered she had 'scant respect for British regulations'.[59] After working for just a few days in Coltford she returned to Cong as her sister, Muriel, was suffering from typhoid. Indeed, as Lynn noted, 'there were tremendous representations made by all sorts of people – both loyalists and unionists did their best – because my patients wanted me back.' Before the end of 1916, Lynn returned to her practice in Dublin. She was given permission to remain in Ireland.[60] At this stage, many of those who had been imprisoned in Britain after the Rising were allowed to return home for Christmas. But 'all the unionist people and all my friends said that nobody would ever go near me on account of my appalling conduct.'[61] She was fortunate to have a profession to return to, unlike many of her republican friends who did not have this economic luxury. However, she was concerned about those who suffered economically because of their involvement in the Rising.

Clearly the few weeks of disruption in Dublin, and elsewhere, during the Rising, had not only disturbed businesses but also deprived many of their income. Furthermore, those involved in the Rising were seen as responsible for the upheaval, and some were not allowed to return to work. A shirt factory was started in Liberty Hall. Lynn admitted that ffrench-Mullen was the 'prime mover in this. She worked it for all she was worth. The girls did not turn out to be a success. I think they wanted proper supervision.'[62] As vice-president of the Irish Women's Workers' Union, Lynn would have been aware of the difficult working conditions facing many women. This union was greatly influenced by Connolly's views on the organisation of labour and was linked to the ICA.

Lynn's attempt to provide employment is indicative of her great concern for others. This was linked to her intense spirituality. She was particularly concerned about the adverse effects of prison on the dependants of prisoners. Her philanthropy and Christianity merged in the provision of relief for the families of republicans. Her friend Kathleen Clarke was particularly involved in the Volunteer Dependants' Fund. Women were seen as especially suited to philanthropy, and Kathleen Clarke distributed large sums of money (over £3,000, it was suggested) after the Rising.[63] In *The Resurrection of Ireland*, Michael Laffan admits that the executive of the Irish National Aid and Volunteer Dependants' Fund disbursed over £138,000 between 1917 and 1920 and that the auditing of the accounts was 'managed as efficiently as the charitable work itself'. Yet he suggests that the 'Prisoners' Aid Society was a charitable rather than a political organisation'. However, Laffan does not depoliticise the organisation entirely as it was 'managed by separatists, in particular the wives and widows of imprisoned or executed rebels'.[64] This work gave women indirect political power, since they decided who would receive aid. Furthermore, the provision of financial support cemented the commitment of relations and friends of those interned.

By early January 1917 Lynn was settled back to her routine at 9 Belgrave Road, in Rathmines. She was exhausted by the previous few months and departed for her spiritual home, County Wicklow.[65] In March she spent time with the Daly family in Limerick, relatives of Kathleen Clarke.[66] By the summer of 1917, many of the republican prisoners were released from various British jails. Characteristically, she simultaneously welcomed Constance Markievicz's return to Ireland and took a swipe at the monarchy: 'Madam's homecoming, crowds greater than ever turned out for royalty.' Three days later she was at Bodenstown, County Kildare, the resting place of Theobald Wolfe Tone, the eighteenth-century republican activist: 'went to Bodenstown, great day, much enthusiasm, Madam spoke.'[67] Tone's vision of a secular republic, without sectarian divisions, provided a model for many. Furthermore, as a Protestant patriot, he was particularly attractive for Lynn. When appealing to the electorate in the 1920s, Lynn explained that she was 'a follower of Tone'.[68]

With republicanism, however, came despair. On 25 September she wrote, 'Thomas Ashe died in Mater while my finger on his pulse. Dev. came at night & he and Emer [Molony] went to Bruagh [sic].'[69] Lynn's finger was on the pulse of nationalists. Her medical expertise, as well as her political commitment, gave her access to the leading nationalists of the period. Thomas Ashe had been force-fed in Mountjoy while on hunger strike. His funeral galvanised nationalists.[70] When de Valera was elected president of Sinn Féin at their Árd Fheis (major gathering) at the Mansion House in Dublin on 25 October, Lynn wrote in her diary that night: 'Meeting congratulating Bolsheviks, Maeve [Maud Gonne MacBride] spoke well, Round Room packed, 2 overflows & street meeting.'[71]

SINN FÉIN

Lynn became a member of the Sinn Féin executive in 1917. This had been no easy task as there were over 100 candidates. At the 1917 Sinn Féin convention, four women were elected to the twenty-four person executive.[72] De Valera was elected on the first count and he became the president of Sinn Féin; Arthur Griffith was vice-president. Lynn received 423 votes, and was the twelfth person elected. Michael Collins, with 340 votes, was the last to be elected.[73] The presence of Lynn and Markievicz was significant later as there were serious attempts to dilute the radical nature of the revolution. Moreover, while the Sinn Féin movement was 'vague', it was an 'organised political force'.[74] Hence, it was important that the views of radical women like Lynn were represented. In May 1917 Lynn spoke along with Arthur Griffith, one of the founders of Sinn Féin, and Count Plunkett, at a mass meeting in the Mansion House which demanded prisoner of war status for Markievicz and her fellow prisoners.[75]

As a very active member of Cumann na dTeachtaire, or the Sinn Féin League of Women Delegates, Lynn's views on the organisation of a new Ireland were articulated.[76] This group of politically active women was crucial in keeping women's rights to the fore in Sinn Féin, and Lynn was a vocal member of the Cumann.

It is clear from the minutes of Cumann na dTeachtaire that these women had no intention of being sidelined in Sinn Féin. Ffrench-Mullen was secretary of the Cumann and, on occasion, Lynn stood in for her. The committee emphasised equal rights from the beginning and insisted on women being represented on the executive committee of Sinn Féin.[77] Despite this radicalism, some traditional views regarding women's roles remained. Countess Plunkett, for example, was not noted for her radicalism. Even Lynn wanted women in charge of what were seen as women's responsibilities. She suggested that women were needed 'in dealing with such questions as the food question.' The Cumann eventually decided that Kathleen Clarke, Áine Ceannt, Jennie Wyse Power, Helena Molony, Alice Ginnell and Lynn would represent women on the Sinn Féin executive. They argued that women had shared the risks and difficulties attendant on establishing a republic.[78] Furthermore, the women who were selected to represent the Cumann on the Sinn Féin executive had been prominent in 1916 and could be relied on to represent the views of women.

On 17 September 1917 the Cumann met in Lynn's home and she chaired the meeting. Lynn, as a member of the executive, offered to help draft a resolution to be brought to the Sinn Féin executive. It lay stress on the fact that in the Sinn Féin organisation 'men' is understood to mean 'men and women', and men and women should be mentioned in all speeches. On a more optimistic note Lynn 'reported the formation of a Food Committee to look after the food supplies of Ireland'. There were two women on this Food Committee, Lynn and Markievicz, and Lynn emphasised again that this was 'a matter closely concerning women'.[79] It may be suggested that Lynn wanted to bring women into the national domestic sphere, that is the day-to-day affairs of the country. Later in the month, Lynn emphasised equality of opportunity as well as articulating the aspiration that women would be eligible for all offices.[80] At the general meeting of the Committee, which had changed its name to Coiste na dTeachtaire, it was decided to produce leaflets in order to facilitate the political education of women. 'Articles about the woman's point of view' were to be published in local papers, and the possibilities of linking with other women's groups were discussed.[81] Clearly, these women realised that while the insurrection was over, the real work of making the republic a reality lay ahead.

Not surprisingly, Lynn was very concerned about health issues. In a 1917 circular, she suggested that food statistics be compiled in order to avoid famine.[82] She realised that awareness of food shortage would galvanise others. Her comments suggest a mixture of pragmatism and idealism. For example, Lynn and ffrench-Mullen wrote an article urging women to further their political rights, given to them by the 'Republican Proclamation'.[83] At meetings Lynn was frequently concerned with raising awareness about women's rights. She was not alone in this respect. Countess Plunkett suggested that, since new administrative councils were being formed,

> it would be well to consider what activities would be most suited to women and it was agreed that departments or subcommittees dealing with organisation, agriculture, education, poor law, health all called for a large proportion of women. Dr Lynn proposed that each member bring next day a list of women suitable to be proposed for these positions.[84]

Lynn was to present this information to the Sinn Féin executive. Hence, she was an essential link between these Sinn Féin women and the new political order which did not place women's rights at the top of its agenda. Because suffrage was not seen as important, these women made their usefulness apparent in particular areas, such as health and welfare. Clearly, these tactics worked initially.

For Lynn, political progress was not matched by domestic bliss. On Christmas Day, 1917 she wrote: 'With Aunt F [Florence, Lynn's mother's sister], a happy day, tho' lonely, they wont have me still at home.'[85] Her father was so horrified by her activities that he refused to let her return home to Cong. Lynn was greatly distressed at her father's intransigence and she was forced to spend Christmas of 1917 with her aunt in Dublin.

Politically, Lynn was as busy as ever. By January 1918, it was noted that some women had been appointed to Sinn Féin committees because of Cumann na dTeachtaire's 'representations'.[86] However, divisions between different women's organisations were also apparent. At a special meeting, chaired by Lynn and held in her home, Cumann na dTeachtaire decided to send three delegates, Miss Barton, a member of a prominent Wicklow nationalist family, Lynn and ffrench-Mullen, to a suffrage meeting organised by the Irish Women's Suffrage and Local Government Association. Since the passage of the Representation of the People Bill, which gave the vote to women over 30 and men over 21, Cumann na dTeachtaire wanted to 'call a conference of the several suffrage societies in Ireland to consider the future with a view to possible amalgamation & invite each society to send three delegates, who would each be entitled to a vote'. Revealingly, the delegates were 'instructed to withdraw, should anything arise to compromise the Society's [Cumann na dTeachtaire] political principles'.[87] Lynn called this meeting because, like other nationalists, she did not want women's political independence to be sacrificed. However, after a 'long' and 'interesting discussion' (perhaps these words were euphemisms for contentious), Cumann na dTeachtaire, by 9 votes to 4, decided to send three delegates. Lynn and ffrench-Mullen were definite delegates and if Miss Barton could not attend, then she was to be replaced by Miss Shanahan.[88] Clearly, the fissures amongst women's groups between those who wanted independence for Ireland and those who were not committed to republican causes were becoming evident. Lynn wanted to impose her will on the committee, hence her decision to call the meeting in the first place and her chairing of the proceedings. However, all were soon overwhelmed with more pressing political issues which affected the health of the nation.

SINN FÉIN AND HEALTH

Public health was a contentious issue in Ireland. It had profound political implications, because local government was, in theory, responsible for the provision of various services. Furthermore, there was growing concern with prostitution and the increase in venereal disease as troops returned from the front. The British state took an increasing interest in venereal diseases (VD) from the 1910s and treatment centres were established. These centres were seen as part of the prevention strategy associated with the Local Government Board and it was further evidence of the British state's concern with a highly infectious disease.[89] The Sinn Féin women took a particular interest in these issues. Lynn and Countess Plunkett were delegated to represent Cumann na dTeachtaire at a public meeting of the Dublin Watch Committee which was held at the end of January 1918 in the Mansion House.[90] The Dublin Watch Committee was concerned about Dublin prostitution and the fact that the police force was entirely male. While Cumann na dTeachtaire was willing to consider more mundane, if pertinent, issues such as the 'utterly inadequate provision of public lavatories for women in Dublin', the public health impact of VD was frightening.[91] Lynn, as director of Public Health for Sinn Féin, was particularly interested in the political impact of infectious diseases. As in the nineteenth century, prostitutes were seen as responsible for transmitting VD and were incarcerated in the Lock Hospital in Dublin, but soldiers were not incarcerated if they had the disease. Ben Novick, in his work on Irish nationalist propaganda, has argued that 'women were both threatening and threatened, and the discourse of morality, produced putatively for the sake of national decency, must also be seen as being produced as an absolute means of control'.[92] This is a misreading of the *Irish Citizen* and the work of Cumann na dTeachtaire. The *Irish Citizen* was the voice of radical suffragists. The writers in this newspaper were concerned about the public health of both prostitutes and the general population. As an advanced nationalist, Lynn blamed the British Army for the spread of the disease, conveniently forgetting or ignoring the fact that many Irishmen fought in the British Army, including her brother John.[93] In many respects, Lynn's argument paralleled Connolly's views. As a 'practical propagandist he condemned the British Garrison, thus making a political rather than a moral point'.[94] As Novick argues, the 'branding of the garrison soldier as a syphilitic was the ultimate form of rejection and condemnation of British rule in Ireland'.[95] But it was deeper than that. As a nationalist as well as a feminist, Lynn saw the garrison as adding to the misery of Irish people, both by spreading disease and infecting a new generation of children. Furthermore, Novick suggests that the protests against the reintroduction of the Contagious Diseases Act, which would have penalised women with VD, were 'ignored' since they were seen as the problem of the 'British garrison'.[96] This is clearly inaccurate as the impetus for the establishment of St Ultan's was a desire to deal with syphilitic infants.[97]

Lynn's concern is very evident in the first public health circular which the Sinn Féin Public Health Department published in February 1918. Lynn's co-author, Dr Richard Hayes, had been medical officer of the Lusk Dispensary District in north Dublin prior to the Rising, and in 1918 was returned as a Sinn Féin MP for East Limerick.[98] With the return of troops from the front, the spectre of VD loomed. It was therefore decided to 'call together a Conference of Irishwomen's Societies this being a matter on which women of every shade of political opinion could unite in order to discuss the best measures to be adopted to combat this evil'.[99] The pamphlet argued that the responsibility for VD lay with the British Army. Hayes and Lynn demanded that every soldier returning to Ireland be tested for the disease.[100] The disease was a political issue, they argued. Lynn and Hayes insisted that infected soldiers should be 'detained in institutions till pronounced free from contagion as determined by the blood-test'. Finally, they rejected the attempt to 'saddle on Irish Public Boards the responsibility of coping with the evil', since this was the responsibility of the British state.[101] As in her work for Cumann na dTeachtaire, Lynn never lost the opportunity to take a swipe at Britain and the abrogation of its responsibilities. One month after the publication of the pamphlet, a conference on VD was held at the Mansion House, on 19 March 1918, under the auspices of Cumann na dTeachtaire.[102] Ultimately, this conference was to result in the establishment of St Ultan's Hospital for Infants.[103]

Allied to the concern with VD and the presence of soldiers was the attempt to impose conscription in Ireland in 1918 when troops were badly needed at the front. The conscription crisis erupted in the spring of 1918 and it galvanised nationalists. Lynn along with other nationalists, Jennie Wyse Power, Agnes O'Farrelly and Alice Stopford Green, were part of the women's protest against conscription.[104] On 9 June 1918, during Women's Day, women were enjoined to 'stand by your countrymen in resisting conscription'. Cumann na dTeachtaire rowed in behind the anti-conscription campaign.[105] Indeed it has been argued that 'the roots of the War of Independence lie in the anti-conscription movement.'[106] Hence, Lynn's linking of disease and British policy in Ireland was a clever political move which was designed to increase nationalist discontent.

At the Annual General Meeting of the League of Women Delegates in April 1918, Sinn Féin women such as Lynn, ffrench-Mullen, Markievicz and Molony declared that Cumann na dTeachtaire had been formed to fulfil the 1916 Proclamation and to 'watch the political movements in Ireland in the interests of Irishwomen'. Furthermore, the objects of the League were

to safeguard the practical rights of Irish women
to ensure adequate representation for women in the Republican Government
to urge and facilitate the appointment of women to public boards throughout the country
to educate Irish women in the rights and duties of citizenship[107]

INFLUENZA PANDEMIC

Lynn was 'on the run' between May and October 1918, until the outbreak of the influenza pandemic. A laconic comment in her diary indicates that she narrowly escaped arrest:

> Evg. meeting of Standing Committee [of Sinn Féin]. Heard the whole executive are to be arrested. I went home, went to Dr Dillon's, G [Gun][108] men came while Dr D & I were at the door. He was taken. I walked out & off. Nearly all the others were taken.

It is surely significant that Lynn was not recognised by the authorities. Clearly she was not a recognisable figure and she was therefore able to perform vital tasks while many of her Sinn Féin colleagues were incarcerated. On 18 May she noted the 'whole executive arrested & deported. Myself on the run.'[109] Her activities during that time indicate her resourcefulness:

> I was not able to carry on my practice except with a few patients. I did not go to my own house. I occasionally saw some patients in their own homes. Miss Molony got up a beautiful rig-out for me. I was supposed to be a war widow, with the military badge of my husband's regiment on my coat. I had my hair powdered and dressed up very beautifully in a way that I ordinarily never wore it. I used go to meetings and went about a good deal. I was always very careful to walk slowly and be a little lame. Of course, I was not like that at all.

She was arrested in October 1918 under the Defence of the Realm regulations, since she was acting or 'about to act in a manner prejudicial to the public safety', and was detained at Arbour Hill.[110] As she noted in her diary, 'Arrested early, brought to Rathmines . . . deportation order cancelled, when guaranteed with Lord Mayor, "no politics". . . Plenty pts [patients] fr[om] 5 pm.'[111] Her dairy makes clear how busy she was. On 30 October it was 'Back to work, injected about 250 in all . . . Belfast prisoners bad. Epidemics (Pneumonia Plague) fearful.' O'Neill, the Lord Mayor of Dublin, convinced the authorities that she was needed during the influenza pandemic. Lynn evidently had influential friends. Dr Charles Cameron, the Chief Medical Officer for Dublin, wrote to the Under-Secretary at Dublin Castle in order to have Lynn released.[112] The authorities agreed to release her.[113] Furthermore, she was not averse to making false promises to the authorities. In October 1918 she signed an undertaking to 'take no part in politics, directly or indirectly'. In direct contravention of that, she was involved with the general election in November/December of the same year. Like many republicans she did not recognise British authority and she was more than willing to use her profession in order to lever concessions from the British state.

O'Neill stated that his intervention on Lynn's behalf 'was dictated solely by a desire to render Dr Lynn free to devote her professional services to the medical work in which she is engaged amongst the poor'.[114] Nonetheless, she was monitored carefully and her home was regularly searched though no incriminating material was found. During 1918, Lynn noted the 'Inignie [sic] protest meeting for women prisoners'.[115] Despite these concerns about ill treatment of political prisoners, Lynn was preoccupied with the flu epidemic and was authoritative and forceful in her plans for coping with the crisis. She helped establish a vaccination scheme in Dublin to prevent more people succumbing to the pandemic. In a letter to Arthur Griffith, she outlined her plans and suggested it was 'a worthy object for a grant from the Dáil'. In a comment reflecting the inefficiency of local government, she wrote:

> People say it is the work of the Corporation or L.G.B. [Local Government Board], well, my experience is that the epidemic would be over before they had done considering the matter.[116]

At the Sinn Féin Árd Fheis in April 1919, Lynn read a report on the flu pandemic which warned that 'the factory of the fever is still in full working order in Flanders – I mean the battlefield'. She advocated open windows, with patients situated beside the window, and proper nourishment.[117] It was through local government in the 1920s that Lynn would advocate the amelioration of people's lives through housing schemes and the improvement of medical facilities. In 1919 we can see her frustration with the pedestrian pace of local government reform. She would come to realise that, while it was convenient to blame the First World War for the ills that beset Ireland in the late 1910s, locally elected officials were often as ineffective as national politicians in the provision of practical responses during medical emergencies. Diarmaid Ferriter has suggested that, 'despite the rhetoric of egalitarianism, many public health priorities seem to have been sidelined during what was an overtly political revolution'.[118] However, he fails to realise that health was used to score political points. Furthermore, Lynn was not content to accept the paltry efforts of local government officials.

Because of official reluctance to take practical steps in order to deal with the flu epidemic Lynn was determined to establish a hospital for infants. However, as noted earlier, it was the problems associated with VD that provided the initial impetus for the hospital. Rapidly St Ultan's became a centre for the flu vaccine. The first reference to 37 Charlemont Street, the eventual site of the hospital, was on the 2 November 1918. 'St B'S 8 o/c. All Souls.

Opened depot for injects, 37 Charlemont St Fair number came, pouring day. Did several pts here.'[119] The following day, she 'saw ab[ou]t opening 37 for pts. Willing help fr. C na B [Cumann na mBan] & others.'[120] On 5 November she bemoaned the fact that there were 'hundreds awaiting burial in Glasnevin'. The following day it was 'Another day of battle with disease.' Later she was more optimistic, 'Hospital doing well, getting into good working swing'.[121]

November also saw the end of the First World War and Lynn's very mild anti-monarchism was evident in her diary. On 11 November, when the armistice was signed, she wrote: 'They say Peace declared, at least it is armistice. Hohenzollerns[122] gone, Republics all round. Much flagwagging here. At night officers on cars & motors attacked by rabble & beaten.'[123] She was too optimistic about the fall of all monarchies. Comically, she declared, 'Labour meeting in Albert Hall "Buckingham Palace to Let".'[124]

Her home was available for political refugees: 'Maeve[125] evading detectives, arrived here [with] Iseult' her daughter.[126] Despite all the political activity, Lynn remained committed to her patients, many of whom were political activists. At the end of November, she had a 'Terribly anxious day with Mrs C[aitlín] Bruagh [sic],[127] stayed in hosp. till 7 a.m. Dr Crofton hurrying up with vaccine.'[128] Lynn also hinted that she was considering the establishment of an infants' hospital: 'Dr Chisholme of Manchester came to see us in 37 & will give useful hints.' Dr Catherine Chisholm was an honorary physician at the Manchester Babies' Hospital as well as Medical Inspector at Manchester High School for Girls. She had published articles on the 'Medical Inspection of Girls in Secondary Schools' and on 'Menstrual Molimina in Girls' in the *Journal of Obstetrics and Gynaecology*.[129] According to Lynn, Chisholm was pleased with St Ultan's.[130] Undoubtedly Lynn and her colleagues learned from Chisholm's experience. Despite Lynn's political distaste for Britain, she was happy to learn from British medicine.

By December 1918 it is clear that Lynn was very excited about Sinn Féin's surge in popularity. Many of their candidates were returned unopposed to Westminster, but, as nationalists, they refused to take their seats. On polling day, 14 December, when seventy-three Sinn Féin candidates were elected to sit in parliament, she wrote: 'memorable day for Ireland. We all hope. May our women's vote be used for the good.' Lynn wanted women to have a say in the running of the new nation. Later, Lynn 'went to Aonach [Fair] in evg. It was very nice & I saw many friends.' The annual Aonach was held in the Mansion House. It was an occasion to display and sell Irish-made goods, plus it was a chance for old friends to meet before Christmas.

Despite Lynn's political friendships, she endured friction with her family. One week before Christmas, she asked, 'When shall I go home again for Christmas?'[131] She spent Christmas with her aunt Florence 'again, very happy, quiet day'. Lynn would have preferred to be with her family in Mayo for Christmas, but her father would not allow her to return home. This personal split would be rectified before her father's death in 1923. Despite the ill feeling caused by her political activity amongst her family, Lynn remained committed to Sinn Féin. At the end of December, at Sinn Féin headquarters on Harcourt Street, when the election results were announced, there was 'great joy everywhere'.[132] What would the New Year bring? It was one matter to win the popular vote, but the difficult task of governing, in a provisional sense, posed a greater challenge.

WAR OF INDEPENDENCE

Despite her commitment to St Ultan's Lynn consolidated her political profile through Sinn Féin activity.[133] As vice-president of Sinn Féin she regularly attended the Standing Committee meetings of the party.[134] When the first Dáil met in 1919, her assessment was that it 'was all that it should be, simple, solemn, impressive – a great voice, God grant a continuance to the end!'[135] However, war brought more grief than solemnity. Lynn's home was raided by the British authorities. She was on call during the raid which yielded no guns, only cigarettes, chocolates, a syringe, a small hot water bottle and 'an embroidered lace collar'.[136] Despite these intrusions, Lynn sustained her activism.

At the Sinn Féin Árd Fheis in April 1919 she submitted a report on the influenza pandemic, noting that the disease was partly the result of the recent war. Her report was adopted. It makes clear her fanaticism for fresh air. She obviously wanted patients outdoors as much as possible. 'Plenty of fresh air is absolutely necessary; patients in rooms with windows and doors open do well'. This seems unwise for a flu victim. 'The English and French have left millions of men and horses to rot unburied where they fell ... the poisonous matter from millions of unburied bodies is constantly rising up into the air, which is blown all over the world by winds.'[137] Clearly germs do not recognise political or geographical boundaries, yet Lynn's advice was tinged with a political ideology. She used medicine to attack the victors of the First World War. The war was blamed for spreading the deadly virus. Furthermore, once the war had ceased there was no effort to cleanse the killing fields of Europe. Lynn therefore blamed the Allies for spreading disease.

In May 1919, Lynn's popularity was confirmed when she was the second person elected, after George Nesbitt, to the fourteen-person Sinn Féin Standing Committee.[138] This committee provided the party with a 'sense of direction'.[139] Given her prominence in public health matters, she was a well-known figure in Sinn Féin circles. Her pamphlet on public health was sent to Dr William Walsh, the nationalistic Roman Catholic Archbishop.[140] Furthermore, she had both the time and the money to devote to various meetings. Fluent in German and French, as well as Irish, she was able to keep abreast of events outside Ireland in the aftermath of the war.

Lynn was very aware of international political developments. During the Versailles Treaty negotiations, like many nationalists she hoped Ireland's voice would be heard. 'Clemenceau [the French Prime Minister] to decide about our representation at Peace Conference. May he do the Right! [sic] At any rate we are a burning question all over the globe now, wherever Irish are and where are they not? & all demand Freedom for their Motherland.'[141] The aspiration that Ireland could take her place amongst the 'small nations of the earth' was to flounder due to the geo-political aims of large nations like Britain. Like many republicans, Lynn placed great hope in the example of the United States, which successfully rebelled against Britain in the eighteenth century. She described 4 July 1921 as 'our great Independence Day', and she wore the US flag as she prayed for Irish liberty in St Ann's Church on Dawson Street, while a couple of doors away in the Mansion House de Valera and Griffith were seeking a political solution to Ireland's difficulties.[142] They were in the Dáil asserting Ireland's right to independence. However, Lynn was to be disappointed when she did not see the establishment of an Irish republic.

It is not surprising, therefore, that the Treaty negotiated in December 1921, which heralded the end of the War of Independence, should agitate Lynn. '"Peace" terms but such a peace! Not what Connolly & Mallin & countless others died for . . . better war than such a peace', she fumed. Later she pronounced that 'our shackles are being refastened'.[143] The reaction of certain women to the Treaty has attracted a lot of historiographical comment. Tom Garvin has been particularly critical of republican women like Lynn. He has even argued that

> women had a certain psychological hold over men. De Valera's relationship of mutual dependence with Cathal Brugha, Mary MacSwiney, Austin Stack and the prominent 'republican women' was curious: an alliance of the steely political purpose of one man and the aggression, hysterical energy and the rage of the rest.

Furthermore, Mary MacSwiney is accused of terrorising the men into voting against the Treaty.[144] Discounting the deeply sexist linking of 'hysteria' and women, Garvin's assertions have absolutely no basis in fact or evidence. Women are a convenient scapegoat. When Tom Garvin suggested that men were motivated by hysteria, Caitriona Clear asked, 'what motivated the men, womb envy?'[145] The emotive language used by MacSwiney and Lynn reinforced the view that women were irrational, but they did not have a monopoly on resentment. Jason Knirck has argued that the republican women were 'rational political actors attempting to speak for, and articulate the interests of, their constituencies'. Assertions that the women were 'emotional' and 'irrational' were simply an attempt to 'undermine' the women.[146]

CIVIL WAR

Lynn's dismay with the Treaty was all too evident. She described those in favour of the Treaty as 'time servers'. Politicians such as Craig, Collins and Churchill were a 'pretty trio'.[147] They were the representatives of Northern Ireland, the Irish Free State and Britain. Lynn was convinced that the republic had been lost. After all, a slight majority had voted for the Treaty. Furthermore, the fact that the king's representative in Ireland, the viceroy, was Tim Healy, whom she saw as a traitor, irked her even more. He had accelerated Parnell's fall from power in the 1890s, now he benefited from the establishment of a new state which was not a republic. 'Tim Healy cost country £38,000 a year, not bad for one man', she sarcastically noted.[148] She saw the victorious pro-Treatyites as imperialist. 'KO'H [Kevin O'Higgins] and Cosgrave [the leader of the anti-treaty party] go to Imperial Conference, just what they're fit for.'[149]

In July and August of 1921, when the pro- and anti-Treatyites were at war, Lynn was based in Waterford and Tipperary. She may have been asked to go to Tipperary which saw a lot of military activity during the early 1920s. Her medical expertise would have been vital. Clearly she was willing to countenance violence in the pursuit of a political dream. This is hardly surprising as she was sympathetic to militant methods as a suffragette. The demands of war were evident from one entry: 'A long day with little food & no rest last night or to-day. We beat off enemy 3 times, heavy fighting along 25 mile front.'[150] With Collins' death later that month, Lynn uncharitably suggested he was 'beloved of a certain set'.[151] Indeed, in common with many republicans, Lynn transferred her criticisms of the British in Ireland to the Free Staters. She was particularly vocal about prisoner maltreatment at the hands of the Irish Free State.[152] Furthermore, she was very critical of the treatment of her anti-treaty friends.

In political terms Lynn was a loser after the Treaty, though she was not to suffer greatly economically. Cumann na nGaedheal, who won the pro-Treaty democratic mandate, sought to curb the power of rebellious republicans like Lynn. Early in 1923, Lynn visited Lausanne in Switzerland with a fellow republican, Kathleen

O'Brennan. Because of her republican activities, Lynn was still monitored carefully. For example, while she was in Switzerland, her house was searched.[153] O'Brennan and Lynn presented a petition on behalf of the Irregulars, as the anti-Treaty group was known, to the International Red Cross Committee.[154] However, the International Red Cross was wary of supporting republicans. Ador, the President of the Red Cross, explained to Kathleen O'Brennan that the refusal of republicans to recognise the Free State meant that the Red Cross was reluctant to intervene in a 'delicate' situation.[155]

Lynn was on the general council of the Irish White Cross and Kathleen Clarke was the honorary secretary. This group also included clergymen and the future historian of the Irish Republic, Dorothy Macardle.[156] It was established in 1920 to fund the victims of the Irish War of Independence. For example, it funded children's education since many were fatherless due to political troubles. As late as 1932, it was noted that the American Red Cross had given £100,000 and the pope had donated £5,000 to the Irish White Cross.[157] Áine Ceannt was secretary of the Irish White Cross and like Lynn she would travel on behalf of republicans so that their cause could be promulgated and funds collected. The *Irish Press* suggested that Ceannt presided 'like a particularly loving godmother, over the destiny of children whose fathers fell or were disabled in the seven years of struggle. Among them are many to whom the six county pogrom of 1920–1922 brought sorrow and bereavement.'[158] The political possibilities of philanthropy were promoted by these peripatetic patriots. Kathleen O'Brennan, Áine Ceannt's sister, Kathleen Clarke and Lynn were involved in the Women Prisoners' Defence Association which presented a petition in 1923 to the Congress of the United States on the conditions of republican prisoners. They calculated that there were over 11,000 republican prisoners in jail, 'including mothers' and they sought 'prisoner of war treatment' for them.[159] Louise Ryan suggests that there were over 300 women in Kilmainhan prison.[160] However, the new Irish state was reluctant to release prisoners whom it saw as a threat to the new state. Lynn and Mary MacSwiney wrote an emotive letter to the Free State government from Sinn Féin headquarters about female prisoners. They suggested that if a man 'kept animals' in the conditions that prisoners endured 'he would be prosecuted'. Damningly, they suggested that Kevin Barry's family endured further misery. He was tortured and executed by the British. His sister, Eileen Barry was tortured in the North Dublin Union. 'Tragedy is inevitable and cannot be averted unless you act at once', they concluded.[161] The efforts of these republicans indicate their willingness to enlist international aid and their desire to promote their cause outside Ireland.

Lynn was aware of international socialist movements, which worked for the amelioration of the conditions of people everywhere. She saw Lenin's death as a great 'loss'.[162] Later, like many other socialists, she failed to see the human rights abuses of the soviet system. She attended Friends of Soviet Russia meetings which were patronised by other republican socialists. For example, in September 1930 the Friends of Soviet Russia invited four Russian workers to visit Ireland. The reception committee included Lynn, ffrench-Mullen, Mrs Cruise O'Brien, Peadar O'Donnell and Frank Ryan. Helena Molony and Hanna Sheehy Skeffington were committee members of the Friends of Soviet Russia.[163]

Lynn's refusal to accept the democratic views of the majority and her inflexibility regarding the legacy of 1916 is evident in her reaction to Sean O'Casey's play, *The Plough and the Stars*, which questioned the blood sacrifice of 1916. The play was disrupted by republican protests. O'Casey's plays exposed the irrelevance of the revolution. Socially Lynn would have sympathised with O'Casey but politically she was unwilling to criticise Pearse's nationalism. As usual, Lynn's diary articulates her emotions: 'We showed what we thought of the Plough & the Stars, it is a horrible travesty on Easter Week.' Later she complained that O'Casey had a 'filthy mind'.[164] As in all civil wars, former friends became enemies. This protest was to become part of theatre history. Christopher Morash presents a compelling picture of a 'night at the theatre'. 'Sighle Humphreys began hissing from the back of the pit', and she was one of several 'experienced agitators and organisers' who made their views known. Morash then suggests that the republican writer Rosamund Jacob recorded 'heated arguments over the play in the Radical Club, where on 20 February Kathleen Lynn read a paper "all against the play"'.[165] However, Jacobs wrote that it was 'A. Lynn' not K. Lynn who presented the paper to the Radical

Club. This is most likely Alexander Lynn who was a member of the Friends of Soviet Russia and no relation of Kathleen Lynn.[166]

POST CIVIL WAR

Margaret MacCurtain has suggested that 'Irish women in post-revolutionary Ireland did not make the political traditions: they inherited them from fathers, husbands and brothers.'[167] Lynn was an exception here, as in many other ways. In 1923 Lynn was elected to the Dáil for Dublin, on the Sinn Féin ticket. However, like all the anti-Treaty republicans, she refused to take her seat. In total, 44 republicans were elected and the governing party, Cumann na nGaedheal, had 63 successful candidates. Lynn was vice-president of Sinn Féin and in February 1923 there was a meeting at the Mansion House which sought to re-organise the party. Lynn told the alleged attendance of 2,000 that the aims of Sinn Féin had not changed. Its 'first and principal object was to secure the international recognition of the existing Irish Republic'. The 'republic is very much alive', Lynn pronounced. She also alluded to the arrest of Sinn Féin activists and the fact that these arrests were not being 'reported in the press. Things are being done on the quiet, and we are here to let you know that the so-called Free State is out to stop these activities of Sinn Féin.' The loss of the political battle was not taken lightly by Lynn and her political friends.[168] During the summer of 1923, the Sinn Féin Re-Organising Committee held an Árd Fheis in order to reactivate former Cumainn, or clubs. Lynn was a member of this committee and she chaired the June meeting which sought to 'secure the recognition of Ireland as an independent Irish Republic'.[169]

SURVIVING THE PEACE

Through her political activity after the Civil War one can see Lynn's interests and concerns. At the Sinn Féin Árd Fheis in 1926, when Lynn was a member of the Standing Committee, she suggested that the 'underfed are always so enervated as to be incapable of action'. She urged every member of a Sinn Féin club 'to help any scheme in his or her area for feeding the people, schemes for feeding of school children, penny dinners, etc.' Furthermore, she encouraged the establishment of 'public health utility societies to promote building in those districts where the housing problem is acute.' As a medical practitioner with a social conscience, Lynn was very aware of economic deprivation which had been acerbated by the political upheaval of the previous decade. Finally, and characteristically, Lynn announced in the Sinn Féin Programme:

> Recognising that in the education of the young lies the only sure foundation of Irish liberty, steps [should] be taken in every area to establish classes for the children to instruct them in the history of their country and particularly of their own countryside and its heroes.[170]

By the mid 1920s, with Sinn Féin still in the political doldrums with no parliamentary representation, there were moves to form a new political party to represent the anti-Treaty side. There is a strong sense of the political strain in her diaries, where she mentions the 'awful feeling of antagonism'. She did not want to enter the Free State parliament. The 'Devites', as she called them, were 'determined' to enter parliament.[171] Ultimately, Lynn did not join the Fianna Fáil party when it was formed in 1926 because she felt it did not remain loyal to the principles enunciated in 1916. She paid the political price for her independence and was soundly defeated in the general election of 1927, when Fianna Fáil established itself as the second largest political party in the state behind the anti-Treaty Cumann na nGaedhael. Lynn refused to join Fianna Fáil because they did not fulfil her aspirations for a political party.

Her 1927 general election poster makes clear her political perspective. Lynn cited major political figures as role models. She was, 'a follower of Wolfe Tone and James Connolly believing with them that *complete separation from the British Empire* is the only way of achieving an honourable and permanent peace for Ireland'. Understandably, Lynn quoted from the Proclamation of 1916 with its resonant call for equality: 'Under a Republican form of Government this can best be accomplished.' Idealistically, she sought to abolish all privileges: status would be earned by 'personal service to the community'. However, given her middle-class background Lynn was one of the fortunate few to have a well-paid profession. She did not always recognise the important work performed by her own servants. Characteristically, she asserted that 'the child is the Nation's most precious possession, [hence] proper provision should be made to enable the mother to bring up her fatherless family'.[172] In conclusion, she reasserted her commitment to Tone's separatism: 'the aim of all true patriots must be that of Wolfe Tone – "to break the connection with England, the never-failing source of all our political evils." That I will be constant to this aim and ceaseless in my efforts to secure it, my fidelity to the Republican cause in the past, and my refusal to compromise in the present, must be my guarantee.'[173]

Lynn's ultimate political failure was her refusal to compromise. She finished at the bottom of the poll in the 1927 election. Fidelity to the republican cause may have garnered political status in the 1910s, but it would not win elections in times of peace. Lynn was philosophical in defeat, however; 'God knows best.'[174] Nonetheless, when the five Sinn Féin TDs favoured entering the Dáil, she 'immediately repudiated it'.[175] By the autumn of 1927 she was clearly becoming tired of the 'weary round of vituperation, one longs for higher ideals,' or the pursuit of a republic. Yet, she was willing to speak at an anti Imperial meeting a month later.[176] Like most republicans, she was intensely antagonistic towards the Empire.

LOCAL GOVERNMENT AND PUBLIC HEALTH

Given her political prominence, it is not surprising that Lynn was elected as a member of Rathmines and Rathgar Urban District Council in 1920 and served for ten years. This Council was unusual in that it boasted several prominent female members, such as ffrench-Mullen, Áine Ceannt, Hanna Sheehy Skeffington, and Mary Kettle, who later chaired the Council, the first female to do so in Ireland. The latter three were widows, and Kettle was particularly interested in the provision of widows' pensions. Rosamund Jacob confided to Sheehy Skeffington that 'nearly all the respectable women in Dublin seem to have got in . . . I hope you'll get some support now in the corporation for sensible doings, though I suppose most of the Sinn Féin men will be just as hopeless about doing anything for the benefit of women as the old crowd were.' Jacob's brother Tom thought that 'Rathmines won't know itself with Dr Lynn & Miss ffrench-Mullen . . . helping to rule its destinies.'[177] These energetic women did not always agree, but Lynn was consistent throughout the decade in her concern for public health improvements. At the Annual General Meeting 30 January 1920, Lynn's first meeting, she was elected unanimously onto the Public Health Committee. She was also elected to the Building Committee, being aware of the close connections between poor housing and ill health.[178] That evening she exulted in her diary, 'we had a lively time & made the old set see we were not to be trifled with'.[179] In April, Lynn was elected to the Rathmines and Pembroke Joint Hospital Board. Throughout the year Lynn was a regular attendee at the various meetings, but the following year, at the height of the War of Independence, she missed several meetings during the summer.

Nonetheless, Lynn was an active councillor. In May 1921 she represented the Council on the National League of Health. In July, she was instrumental in ensuring that when doctors conducted health visits, 'infant consultations' also took place. Lynn also became a member of the Child Welfare Committee. This activity dovetailed with her work in St Ultan's where she negotiated with local politicians in order to improve the provision of welfare facilities such as babies' clubs.[180]

In November 1924 Lynn and ffrench-Mullen tried to have Hanna Sheehy Skeffington co-opted onto the Committee, but they were unsuccessful. The following year, Lynn tried to have Mary Kettle elected as chairman, yet again this was unsuccessful. Meanwhile, in 1925, Lynn was elected onto the Housing and Building Committee, the Public Health Committee and the Child Welfare Committee. She was also one of the Rathmines Representatives on the Rathmines and Pembroke Joint Hospital Board. It is clear from their activities on the Council that Lynn and Kettle were particularly concerned about economic deprivation. In November

1926 Kettle proposed and Lynn seconded a motion that school meals be provided in the child welfare centre. This motion was carried unanimously. The Council was particularly concerned about hunger and the lack of fuel.[181] It is surprising that this issue was not contentious because the provision of school meals was controversial in the 1940s and welfare was distributed along denominational lines.[182] However, not all were as concerned as Lynn about deprivation. Dr Goulding, a fellow councillor, suggested that child welfare was not needed in Rathmines. Lynn gasped at the 'horror of a mind like his'.[183] Certainly Rathmines was not the worst affected area. In the Rathmines township, close to Charlemont Street where St Ultan's was located, there were some very deprived areas. Dublin had the worst infant mortality rate in the country. At a national level, in 1926, 74 infants in every thousand did not reach their first birthday.[184]

Lynn also represented the Council abroad, as she was a delegate in 1929 to the Royal Institute of Public Health in Zurich. Lynn reported to the Council her impressions of the congress and this report was sent to the Minister for Local Government and Public Health.[185] The following year the RRUDC was integrated into Dublin Corporation and Lynn's formal political career ceased. However, the activities she was most associated with on the Council continued through her work at St Ultan's.

CONCLUSION

In a poem by Deborah Webb,[186] dedicated to Lynn, in May 1919, Webb advocated active patriotism:

> Loving thy mother country well,
> Yet pray avoid the patriot's cell,
> Needed in all thy martial might,
> Nature allied, disease to fight.[187]

St Ultan's Hospital for Infants sought to nurture future citizens. A Sinn Féin election poster declared that 'women in an Irish parliament are absolutely necessary to keep a watchful eye on your interests. Sinn Féin has translated words into deeds by nominating women candidates for Irish constituencies.'[188] Despite the optimism that Sinn Féin would treat women fairly, the 1920s were to see that hope fade. Clearly, a small and dynamic group of women who were highly politicised could assert the importance of women in national politics. In the case of Lynn, as suggested at the beginning of this chapter, professional inequality was a politicising experience. Lynn's philosophy and philanthropy found fulfilment in medicine, not politics. Her professional skills were vital in the aftermath of 1916. She was to act as a medical officer during and after the Rising and she exposed the unhealthy conditions of prisoners.

In some ways, Lynn confined herself to traditional areas of female endeavour, with her concern for health and education. Many political women, after the first flush of revolution and political activity in the early twentieth century, devoted their later careers to maternal feminism, that is feminism which emphasised the importance of welfare and the rights of women and children. The League of Women Delegates is a good example of this kind of activity. While Lynn and her colleagues wished to politicise women, ultimately they were to find fulfilment in the maternal work of St Ultan's and frustration in the messy work of political life. They wanted to make women aware of their rights and responsibilities as citizens in the newly emerging state.[189] Lynn did not have the impact on national politics she desired and deserved. The fact that she put herself forward as a candidate in 1927 suggests that she wanted a political career. The suffrage movement, which initially politicised Lynn, was successful. In 1918 a limited franchise was introduced for women in Britain and Ireland. Women over thirty who were property owners or university graduates were entitled to vote. As a graduate of the Royal University of Ireland, Lynn received the vote. In 1922 the Irish Free State introduced equal suffrage.

By 1930 Lynn was no longer a TD or an urban district councillor, and she devoted the rest of her career to St Ultan's. Through medicine she was to articulate her vision for a secular republic. The intense political activity of the 1910s and '20s gave her national prominence but she faded from the public eye in the 1930s.

However, she never lost her radical aspirations. Lynn would cherish the children of the nation in St Ultan's.

NOTES

1. In 1912 James Connolly wrote that 'Ireland has today within her bosom two things that must make the blood run with riotous exaltation in the veins of every lover of the Irish race – a disenchanted working class, and the nucleus of a rebellious womanhood.' James Connolly, *Irish Worker*, Christmas 1912, cited in W.K. Anderson, *James Connolly and the Irish Left* (Dublin, Portland and Melbourne, 1993), p. 16.
2. The executive committee consisted of 49 people, while Anna Haslam was the honorary secretary. *Report of the Executive Committee of the Irish Women's Suffrage and Local Government Association for 1902* (Dublin, 1902), p. 3, see annual reports up to 1916.
3. Finn, 'Women in the medical profession', p. 116.
4. Ruane, 'Lynn', p. 68; Sylvia Pankhurst to Lynn, 7 Dec. 1916, in Madeleine ffrench-Mullen file in Allen Library, Dublin. Sylvia Pankhurst (1882–1960) was a 'passionate socialist': see Cheryl Law, *Suffrage and Power: The Women's Movement, 1918–1928* (London and New York, 1997), p. 240.
5. Mary Cullen, 'Anna Maria Haslam (1829–1922)', in Mary Cullen and Maria Luddy (eds), *Women, Power and Consciousness in Nineteenth-Century Ireland: Eight Biographical Studies* (Dublin, 1995), pp. 161–96, p. 182.
6. Rosemary Cullen Owens, *Smashing Times: A History of the Irish Women's Suffrage Movement: 1889–1922* (Dublin, 1984 and 1995), pp. 51–3.
7. Brother Allen Papers, Lynn's first statement, Allen Library, Dublin. This is an exact copy of Lynn's statement to the Bureau of Military History. My thanks to Frances Clarke of the Military Archives for clarifying this.
8. Mary Cullen, 'Anna Maria Haslam (1829–1922)' in Cullen and Luddy (eds), *Women, Power and Consciousness in Nineteenth-Century Ireland*, pp. 161–96.
9. *Irish Citizen*, December 1913, cited in Louise Ryan (ed.), *Irish Feminism and the Vote: An Anthology of the Irish Citizen Newspaper, 1912–1920* (Dublin, 1996), p. 40. This book is an excellent source for the *Irish Citizen* newspaper, an influential organ of feminists and suffragists, as well as the mouthpiece of the Irish Citizen Army.
10. Obituary of Lynn, *Irish Press*, 15 Sept. 1955.
11. Brother Allen Papers, Lynn's first statement, Allen Library, Dublin.
12. For an excellent regional discussion of Cumann na mBan, see Marie Coleman, "They also served": the Role of Cumann na mBan in the War of Independence – the Evidence from County Longford', in *PaGes. Postgraduate Research in Progress*, UCD Arts Faculty, Volume 5, 1998, pp. 31–42; the foundation of Inghinidhe na hÉireann is described in Maria Luddy (ed.), *Women in Ireland, 1800–1918: A Documentary History* (Cork, 1995 and 1999), pp. 300–9.

13 Margaret Ward, *Unmanageable Revolutionaries: Women and Irish Nationalism* (Dublin, 1989).
14 Cited in obituary of Lynn, *Irish Times*, 15 Sept. 1955.
15 Austen Morgan, *James Connolly: A political Biography* (Manchester, 1988), p. 144.
16 Anderson, *James Connolly and the Irish Left*, p. 21.
17 Lynn's first statement, Allen Library, Dublin.
18 Lynn's first statement, Allen Library, Dublin.
19 James Connolly, *The Reconquest of Ireland* (Dublin, Irish Transport and General Workers Union, 1934, first published in 1915), pp. 289–90.
20 Susan L. Mitchell, *Red-Headed Rebel: Poet and Mystic of the Irish Cultural Renaissance* (Dublin, 1998), p. 208. Mitchell would have known Lynn through the Irish Guild of the Church, pp. 175–6.
21 *Irish Citizen*, 15 Feb. 1913.
22 Gladys Evans was forcibly fed for fifty-eight days; Rosemary Cullen Owens, *Smashing Times: A History of the Irish Women's Suffrage Movement, 1889–1922* (Dublin, 1984 and 1995), p. 64.
23 Lynn to Hanna Sheehy Skeffington, (no date), HSS Papers MS 21,649, National Library of Ireland (NLI).
24 Palmer to Hanna Sheehy Skeffington, 11 August 1914, HSS Papers MS 22,666 (iv), (NLI).
25 My thanks to Sinéad McCoole for bringing this photograph to my attention. It has been reproduced in Margaret Ward, 'The League of Women Delegates & Sinn Féin' in *History Ireland*, autumn 1996, pp. 37–41; p. 39.
26 LD, 17 March 1916.
27 Alvin Jackson, *Ireland, 1798–1998* (London, 1999), pp. 201–2.
28 Lynn's first statement, Allen Library, Dublin. The ink bottle is in the National Museum, Collins Barracks, Dublin.
29 Lynn's first statement, Allen Library, Dublin.
30 Countess Markievicz, '1916–1926', *Cumann na mBan*, vol. II, no. 10, 1926, pp. 1–3, ILB NLI 94109 P4.
31 Ibid.
32 Speech made by Nora Connolly O'Brien, 3 February 1957, at the opening of the surgical unit in St Ultan's, in de Valera Papers, P150 (de Valera kept a file on Lynn) in UCD Archives. I am grateful to Séamus Helferty for facilitating my access to this file.
33 Lynn's first statement, Allen Library, Dublin.
34 Michael Laffan, *The Resurrection of Ireland: The Sinn Féin Party, 1916–1923* (Cambridge, 1999), p. 48.
35 LD, 25 April 1916.
36 Lynn's second statement, Allen Library. All Lynn quotations are taken from this statement, unless source is cited.
37 LD, 25 and 26 April 1916.
38 Ruth Taillon, *When History was Made: The Women of 1916* (Belfast, 1996) p. 104.

39 Kathleen Clarke, (edited by Helen Litton), *Revolutionary Woman: My Fight for Ireland's Freedom* (Dublin, 1991), pp. 89 and 121.
40 LD, 1 May 1916.
41 Clarke, *Revolutionary Woman*, p. 92.
42 Lynn's second statement, Allen Library.
43 LD, 1 and 2 May 1916.
44 LD, 3 May 1916.
45 LD, 4 and 6 May 1916.
46 LD, 30 April 1916.
47 LD, 6 and 7 May 1916.
48 LD, 8 May 1916.
49 Marie O'Neill, *Grace Gifford Plunkett and Irish Freedom: Tragic Bride of 1916* (Dublin, 2000), pp. 34–50.
50 LD, 9 May 1916.
51 LD, 10 May 1916.
52 Lynn's first statement; LD, 29 April 1916.
53 LD, 8 May 1916.
54 Unfortunately we do not know who these journalists were, they may have been writing for Irish-American newspapers.
55 Lynn's first statement; LD, 12 May 1916.
56 *Freeman's Journal*, 14 June 1916.
57 LD, 17 May 1916.
58 Lynn's first statement, Allen Library.
59 Brian Cusack, Witness Statement, 736, Military Archives, Cathal Brugha Barracks, Dublin.
60 Chief Secretary's Office, T.J.D. Atkinson, Captain of DMP [Dublin Metropolitan Police] to Chief Commissioner of DMP, 13503/16, NAI.
61 Lynn's second statement, Allen Library.
62 Lynn's second statement, Allen Library.
63 Laffan, *The Resurrection of Ireland* p. 67.
64 Ibid., pp. 68, 75 and 66.
65 LD, 1, 13, 14 and 16 Jan. 1917.
66 LD, 17 May 1917.
67 LD, 21 June and 24 June 1917.
68 See discussion of Lynn's 1927 election poster on pp. 51–2.
69 LD, 25 Sept. 1917.
70 The 'Dev' Lynn referred to was Éamon de Valera who would dominate Irish politics for decades. He would become president of Sinn Féin that October. Noted for his charisma and conservatism, he would be a distant admirer of Lynn and she, in turn, had a love-hate relationship with this pragmatic, political animal. Brugha was Cathal Brugha who would be killed in the Civil War of 1921–23.
71 LD, 25 Oct. 1917.
72 Laffan, *The Resurrection of Ireland*. p. 193
73 Tomás Ó Dochartaigh, *Cathal Brugha: A Shaol is a Thréithe* (Dublin, 1969), pp. 63–4.

74 Laffan, *The Resurrection of Ireland* p. 121.
75 Sinn Féin Pamphlet, Item 12, NLI ILB 300, p. 6
76 Margaret Ward, 'League of Women Delegates' pp. 37–41.
77 Minute Book of Cumann na dTeachtaire meeting, 23 July 1917, MS 21,194 (47), NLI.
78 Minute Book of Cumann na dTeachtaire meeting, 30 July 1917, MS 21,194 (47), NLI.
79 Minute Book of Cumann na dTeachtaire meeting, 17 Sept. 1917, MS 21,194 (47), NLI.
80 Minute Book of Cumann na dTeachtaire meeting, 20 Sept. 1917, MS 21,194 (47), NLI.
81 Minute Book of Cumann na dTeachtaire meeting, 26 Oct. 1917, MS 21,194 (47), NLI.
82 Sinn Féin Circular, in Hanna Sheehy Skeffington Papers, MS 8786 (1), NLI. A Sinn Féin Circular was issued from 6 Harcourt Street, their headquarters, on 10 October 1917, which listed Lynn as a member of the Sinn Féin Food Committee.
83 Minute Book of Cumann na dTeachtaire meeting, 20 Sept. 1917, MS 21,194 (47), NLI.
84 Minute Book of Cumann na dTeachtaire meeting, 20 Nov. 1917, MS 21,194 (47), NLI.
85 LD, 25 Dec. 1917.
86 Minute Book of Cumann na dTeachtaire meeting, 15 Jan. 1918, MS 21,194 (47), NLI. We are not told who these women were. Clearly Cumann na dTeachtaire wanted to be represented on Sinn Féin committees, which, in the words of Laffan, were 'the equivalent of government departments', Laffan, *The Resurrection of Ireland,* p. 182. The Sinn Féin Standing Committee minutes in NLI P3269 do not list the members of each department.
87 Minute Book of Cumann na dTeachtaire meeting, 15 Jan. 1918 and 14 Feb. 1918, MS 21,194 (47), NLI.
88 Minute Book of Cumann na dTeachtaire meeting, 14 Feb .1918, MS 21,194 (47), NLI. The following were present at the meeting: 'Countess Plunkett, Mrs Ceannt, Miss Kennedy, Miss Molony, Miss Fitzgerald, Miss Davis, Miss Shanahan, Mrs Clarke, Miss ffrench-Mullen, Miss O'Grady and Mrs Ginnell.'
89 David Evans, 'Tackling the "Hideous Scourge": The creation of venereal disease treatment centres in early twentieth-century Britain', in *Social History of Medicine*, vol. 5, no. 3, December 1992, pp. 413–433. 'In 1917 county councils were given the task of setting up VD clinics under the Public Health Act (Ireland)'; Greta Jones, *'Captain of all these men of death': The History of Tuberculosis in Nineteenth and Twentieth Century Ireland* (Amsterdam and New York, 2001), p. 10. My thanks to the author for giving me a copy of her book.
90 Minute Book of Cumann na dTeachtaire meeting, 26 Feb. 1918, MS 21,194 (47), NLI.

91 Minute Book of Cumann na dTeachtaire meeting, 26 Feb .1918, MS 21,194 (47), NLI.
92 Ben Novick, *Conceiving Revolution: Irish Nationalist Propaganda during the First World War* (Dublin, 2001), p. 150.
93 John Lynn was discharged from the British Army in May 1916, see WO 364/2185/ Service file on John Lynn, in National Archives (PRO) Kew. My thanks to Marie Coleman for locating this file for me.
94 Novick, *Conceiving Revolution* p. 152.
95 NIbid., p. 154.
96 Ibid., p. 156.
97 The establishment of St Ultan's will be discussed in chapter 3.
98 Hayes graduated in medicine in 1905. He was imprisoned in Frongach and Pentonville after 1916. In the 1930s he was to become a prize-winning historian of eighteenth-century Ireland. See Kirkpatrick Biographical Archive, RCPI, *Medical Press and Circular,* 24 May 1916, T*he Times,* 20 Sept. 1917, *Irish Press,* 24 Feb. 1934, *Weekly Irish Times,* 14 Dec. 1940.
99 Minute Book of Cumann na dTeachtaire meeting, 26 Feb. 1918, MS 21,194 (47), NLI.
100 Richard Hayes and Kathleen Lynn, *Public Health Circulars, no. 1,* (Sinn Féin Public Health Department, Dublin, February, 1918).
101 Ibid., p. 4.
102 Minute Book of Cumann na dTeachtaire meeting, 2 April 1918, MS 21,194 (47). NLI.
103 See chapter 3 for the establishment of St Ultan's.
104 Marie O'Neill, *From Parnell to De Valera: A Biography of Jennie Wyse Power, 1858–1941* (Dublin, 1991), p. 104.
105 Robert Barton Scrapbook, unpaginated, MS 5637, NLI.
106 Pauric Travers, *Eamon de Valera* (Dublin, 1994), p. 15.
107 Minute Book of Cumann na dTeachtaire meeting, 2 April 1918, MS 21,194 (47), NLI.
108 G. Men were detectives who concentrated on political crimes.
109 LD, 17 and 18 May 1918.
110 Order under Regulation 14.B of the Defence of the Realm Regulations CO904/207/251, National Archives (PRO), Kew. My thanks to Maria Luddy for copying this material for me.
111 LD, 30 and 31 Oct. 1918.
112 Charles Cameron to Under-Secretary, 31 Oct. 1918, Lynn file CO 904/207/251, PRO Kew.
113 *Evening Mail,* 31 Oct. 1918.
114 Signed undertaking by Lynn, Lynn file CO 904/207, and O'Neill to James McMahon, Under-Secretary for Ireland, 31 Oct. 1918, Lynn file CO 904/207, National Archives (PRO), Kew.
115 LD, 22 Sept. 1918.
116 Lynn to Griffith, no date, but probably November 1918, Allen Library.
117 Sinn Féin Pamphlet, Árd Fheis, 8 April 1919, NLI ILB 300, p. 5.

118 Diarmaid Ferriter, *'Lovers of Liberty?' Local Government in 20th century Ireland* (Dublin, 2001), pp. 136–37; Diarmaid Ferriter, 'Local government, public health and welfare in twentieth-century Ireland', in Mary E. Daly (ed.), *County and Town: One Hundred Years of Local Government in Ireland* (Dublin, 2001), pp. 109–19, p. 110.
119 LD, 2 Nov. 1918.
120 LD, 3 Nov. 1918.
121 LD. 5, 6 and 8 Nov. 1918.
122 The Prussia/Brandenburg royal family (1415–1918).
123 LD, 11 Nov. 1918.
124 LD, 15 Nov. 1918.
125 Maud Gonne MacBride, a committed nationalist, as well as the estranged wife of John MacBride, who had been executed in 1916.
126 Lynn was Iseult's doctor from 1918 until the 1930s; LD, 24 Nov. 1918.
127 Caitlín was Cathal Brugha's wife, she was elected to the Dáil in the 1923 and she shared Lynn's uncompromising republicanism.
128 LD, 26 Nov. 1918.
129 *Medical Directory*, 1919 p. 564.
130 Peter D. Mohr, 'Dr Catherine Chisholm (1879–1952) and the Manchester Babies' Hospital (Duchess of York)', in *Transactions of the Lancashire and Cheshire Antiquarian Society*, vol. 94, 1998, pp. 95–110. My thanks to Conor Ward for giving me this excellent article.
131 LD, 14, 16, 18 and 28, 1918.
132 LD, 28 and 29, Nov.
133 St Ultan's is discussed in chapter 3.
134 Sinn Féin Standing Committee Minute Book (Jan. 1918–May 1919), P3269, NLI.
135 LD, 21 Jan. 1919.
136 Erskine Childers, *Military Rule in Ireland: A series of Eight Articles contributed to the Daily News March – May, 1920* (Dublin, 1920), p. 13. My thanks to Angela Bourke for this reference.
137 Kathleen Lynn, 'Report on Influenza Epidemic, March 1919', in Sinn Féin Election Material, NLI ILB 33, p. 5.
138 Sinn Féin material in Robert Barton Scrapbook, unpaginated, MS 8786 (1), NLI.
139 Laffan, *The Resurrection of Ireland*, p. 176.
140 William Walsh Papers, Lay files, 1918, Dublin Diocesan Archives.
141 LD, 27 June 1919.
142 LD, 4 July 1921.
143 LD, 7 and 8 December 1921.
144 Tom Garvin, *1922: The Birth of Irish Democracy* (Dublin, 1996) p. 96.
145 Caitriona Clear, 'Review of Margaret Ward *The Missing Sex: Putting Women into Irish History*', in *Linen Hall Review*, 1987, p. 81.
146 Jason Knirck, '"Ghosts and Realities": female TDs and the Treaty debate', in *Éire-Ireland*, winter 1997, vol. xxxii, no. 4, pp. 170–94, p. 178.
147 LD, 21 Jan. and 1 April 1922.

148 LD, 8 June 1923.
149 LD, 25 Sept. 1923.
150 LD, 2 August 1922.
151 LD, 23 August 1922.
152 LD, 13 March 1923.
153 Letter from Berne, Switzerland, 19 Jan. 1923, to Minister of External Affairs, Department of An Taoiseach, S.3147, NAI. I am grateful to Gerard McKeown for this reference.
154 R.M. Hodgson, British Commercial Mission, Moscow, to Marquess Curzon of Kedleston, 8 June 1923, which noted that a telegram from the 'Ligue des dammes irlandaises pour la defence des prisonnieres' had been signed by Charlotte Despard, President of the Association, Lynn and O'Brennan secretaries; Dept. of An Taoiseach, S.3147, NAI.
155 Ador to O'Brennan, in Áine Ceannt/Lily O'Brennan Papers, NLI MS Dept., PC661–666, Box 3, file 26. I am grateful to Maria Luddy for alerting me to the extensive Ceannt/O'Brennan Papers, and to Gerry Lyne and Tom Desmond for facilitating my access to them.
156 Áine Ceannt/Lily O'Brennan Papers, NLI MS Dept., PC661–666, Box 4, file entitled, 'Red Cross Material'. My thanks to Nadia Smith, who has written a Ph.D. at Boston College on female historians, for enlightening me on Macardle.
157 *Irish Press*, 28 May 1932, in Ceannt/O'Brennan Papers, NLI MS Dept., PC661–666, Box 4, file marked 'Mrs Eamonn Ceannt'.
158 *Irish Press*, undated, in Ceannt/O'Brennan Papers, NLI MS Dept., PC661–666, Box 4, file 8.
159 Ceannt/O'Brennan Papers, NLI MS Dept., PC661–666, Box 4, Miscellaneous file.
160 Louise Ryan, '"Furies" and "Die-hards"': Women and Irish Republicanism in the Early Twentieth Century in *Gender and History*, vol. 11, no. 2, July 1999, pp. 256–75, p. 269.
161 File on Civil War Prisoners, Dept. of An Taoiseach, S1369–10, NAI. This massive file is indicative of the ill feeling generated by the incarceration of republicans, or Irregulars, as they were known. My thanks to Maria Luddy who alerted me to this file. All of the Dept. of An Taoiseach files that relate to women are accessible on the National Archives website as part of the Women's History Project.
162 LD, 23 Jan. 1924.
163 Communist Activity in the Free State 1929–, NAI, Dept. of An Taoiseach, S5074B.
164 LD, 11 Feb. and 1 March 1926.
165 Christopher Morash, *A History of Irish Theatre 1601–2000* (Cambridge, 2002), pp. 163–70.
166 Rosamund Jacob Diary, 1 January–9 April 1926, NLI MS Dept., Ms 32,582 (47), p. 41.
167 Margaret MacCurtain, 'Women, the vote and revolution', in Margaret MacCurtain and Donncha Ó Corráin (eds), *Women in Irish Society: The Historical Dimension* (Dublin, 1978), pp. 46–57, p. 54.

168 Sinn Féin Re-Organisation Meeting in the Mansion House, 11 Feb. 1923, NLI L.O. P95.
169 Sinn Féin Re-Organising Committee, 4 July 1924, NLI ILB 300 p5; *Sinn Féin*, October 1923.
170 Sinn Féin Clár [Programme] Árd Fheis, 1926, P. 2279, NLI.
171 LD, 10 and 18 March 1926.
172 After the political trauma of the 1919–23 period, some families would have been fatherless. Furthermore, widows and orphans pensions were not introduced until 1935.
173 Lynn's Election Poster, Diary insert, St Ultan's Archives (SUA).
174 LD, 13 June 1927.
175 LD, 22 August 1927.
176 LD, 8 Sept. and 27 Oct. 1927.
177 Rosamund Jacob to Hanna Sheehy Skeffington, 18 Jan. 1920, quoted in Leah Levenson and J.H. Natterstad, *Hanna Sheehy-Skeffington, Irish Feminist* (Syracuse, 1986), p. 133.
178 Minutes of the Rathmines and Rathgar Urban District Council (hereafter RRUDC) are held at the Dublin City Archives, Dublin. Bríd Leahy has extracted all the references to female members and I am very grateful for her help, see Bríd Leahy, *Dublin City Archives: Abstract of political career of Dr Kathleen Lynn as a member of the Rathmines and Rathgar Urban District Council, 1920–1930* (Dublin, 2000). The discussion of Lynn's work on the Council is based on the minutes of the RRUDC.
179 LD, 30 Jan. 1920.
180 Lynn's work in St Ultan's during the 1920s will be discussed in chapter 3.
181 Special Council meeting regarding school children and the lack of fuel due to unemployment, 8 Nov. 1926, RRUDC Minutes, Dublin City Archives.
182 Hilda Tweedy, *A Link in the Chain: The Story of the Irish Housewives Association, 1942–1992* (Dublin, 1992). Providing school meals was seen by some as 'breaking up the sanctity of the home'. David Sheehy, Dublin Diocesan Archivist, suggests that the IHA was seen as a 'threat to national security' by some of the more paranoid members of the clergy.
183 LD, 31 March 1925.
184 Caitriona Clear, *Women of the House: Women's Household Work in Ireland, 1922–1961* (Dublin, 2000), p. 127.
185 Her report is not in the RRUDC archives.
186 Deborah Webb was a Quaker and a friend of Lynn and Hanna Sheehy Skeffington.
187 Webb poem in Lynn Papers, Allen Library.
188 Sinn Féin election poster, NLI ILB 33 P6, item 75.
189 Minute Book of Cumann na dTeachtaire meeting, 30 Jan. 1919 MS 21,194 (47), NLI.

CHAPTER THREE

'A University for Mothers', 1919–30[1]

By the early 1920s, Lynn was a well-known figure. She had gained prominence through her Sinn Féin activities. However, a decade later she had faded from national politics and devoted the rest of her career to 'political philanthropy'. What had brought about this transformation? Social and maternal feminism encouraged politically active women to focus on welfare issues, in particular on women's and children's health. It placed great emphasis on the importance of motherhood and the support of women and children. 'Since the late nineteenth century women's struggles for political and social rights, citizenship, and welfare had been closely linked, and the women's movements had focused more sharply than ever on the needs and interests of lower-class women and on female poverty.'[2] A quiet revolution in public health took place in western Europe in the early twentieth century. However, it has barely been examined in Irish history.[3] Lynn endured a noisy revolution in politics and prepared herself to be part of a noiseless revolution in paediatrics and public health. Through their work in St Ultan's, Lynn and her colleagues were to impinge on many aspects of national life.

The late nineteenth- and early twentieth-century public health and sanitation reform impulses were not unique to Ireland. Internationally, the increasing prominence of politicised women and the focus on citizenship had placed the spotlight on those whose needs the state had neglected. In France, for example, there was a call to provide 'social protection' for all mothers. Furthermore, in the aftermath of an exhausting World War there were increasing concerns about poor population growth. Inevitably, infant mortality became a focus for governments who wished to rejuvenate the nation. Population growth, then, was placed on the political agenda and it forced nations to assess the public health of their people. Ireland was not immune to these concerns. Mokyr has argued that 'the idea that children were worth protecting and nurturing became central to late- nineteenth- and early twentieth-century reformism'. Furthermore, Lynn's life coincided with the bacteriological revolution. The discovery of germs and their role in the spread of infection in the late nineteenth century impacted on the lives of medical professionals. Lynn was fortunate that her career bridged the gap between the sanitation and vaccination movements. However, most of her professional activity took place prior to the introduction of vaccines. Hence, great stress was placed on the elimination of dirt.[4] This greater awareness of disease and germs and the belief that illness could be prevented through maternal vigilance placed grave responsibilities on women. Lynn's medical career was the personification of these concerns. In 1950 she declared:

> The lack of knowledge of the treatment of infants at that time [in the 1910s] was appalling and the attention given to them in the general hospitals was very defective, only surgical cases being treated. No interest was taken in malnutrition and kindred complaints. We considered it high time that this state of affairs should be remedied.[5]

The presence of women on health committees constituted political radicalism. For example, the 1915 Notification of Births Act gave the power to appoint a committee which was 'to include women'. In response to this, the Pembroke Urban Council in Dublin appointed a maternity and child welfare committee, which included poor law guardians, members of the Women's National Health Association (WNHA) and a Medical Superintendent Officer of Health.[6] This link between women and health was not unique to Ireland. The Scandinavian Women's Sanitary Association, which was founded in 1896, and the 'siamese triplets' of the National Association for Women's Suffrage the Association for Women's Rights, and the Women's Sanitary Organisation worked together to improve both the health of the nation, and women's rights.[7] Progressive schools were quick to latch on to the connection between hygiene and women. Alexandra College, Lynn's Alma Mater, linked with Trinity College in establishing a course on Sanitary and Applied Hygiene, in 1908. Dr Katherine Maguire and Dr Ella Webb, who were later to work in St Ultan's, both taught on the course which sought to prepare students for work under the Department of Agriculture and Technical Instruction.[8] Tuberculosis committees also tended to have female members.

That females were seen as particularly important in the drive towards better hygiene, was a notion articulated by Lady Aberdeen, the viceroy's wife. She founded the WNHA in 1907 in order to lower tuberculosis rates. Her 1911 presidential address to the Royal Institute of Public Health was entitled, 'The Sphere of Women in Relation to Public Health'. In order for new medical ideas to be successful, she argued, the 'confidence of the housewives' had to be sought. They would help to 'popularise' new ideas regarding health as they were the people who 'moulded' ideas in the home. Lady Aberdeen wanted to have household science made compulsory for women in university. She suggested that placing domestic science on the curriculum would raise the status of the subject.[9] These views would be echoed by Lynn's colleagues in St Ultan's, some of whom were active in the WNHA. Given their involvement in public health, it is not surprising that female doctors were prominent in the WNHA. Primarily concerned with reducing the frightening TB death rate, it wished to educate the public, particularly women, on health matters. Its interests ranged from hygiene to the distribution of milk and the lowering of the infant mortality rate. The WNHA established dozens of local branches, and travelled the country with medical experts delivering lectures on public health. Their local branches ultimately linked up with nursing groups and child welfare schemes. They established Babies' Clubs and TB dispensaries. The WNHA exerted political pressure to have public health legislation (for example, the 1907 and 1915 Notification of Births Acts) implemented, and they sought funding for child welfare. Sanatoria in Newcastle, County Dublin (Peamount), and Rossclare, County Fermanagh were established by the WNHA to cater for TB patients. As their golden jubilee report noted in 1957, much of the work 'pioneered by the WNHA has been taken over by local and government authorities'.[10]

The work of the WNHA in reducing infant mortality was noted by William Lawson in the *Journal of the Statistical and Social Inquiry Society of Ireland* in 1919. He commented on the cooperation sought between the Infant Aid Society, the WNHA and the Public Health Department of Dublin Corporation. Lawson referred to the reports on the physical welfare of mothers and children by Drs Marion Andrews, Ella Webb, and Alice Barry. They discussed what was being done in Belfast, Dublin, and Cork respectively.[11] Both Webb and Barry worked with Lynn in St Ultan's. It has been suggested, in relation to child welfare, that the First World War brought to 'Ireland the language but not the reality of social reform'.[12] In a sense, the WNHA was filling this gap between rhetoric and reality in the medical world. They initiated a nationwide campaign to spread the gospel of cleanliness. Their travels, from Donegal to Waterford, with a health caravan emblazoned with the motto, 'War on Germs', took on the appearance of an evangelical crusade. The WNHA also produced a journal, *Sláinte*, from 1909. Through it they advertised their varied activities, from lectures to establishing a pasteurised milk depot. The WNHA brought both the language and the reality of sanitary reform to many parts of Ireland. It was not unusual for a combination of aristocratic and professional women to combine their resources in order improve public health. The infant mortality rate of New Zealand was reduced from 8 per cent in 1902 to 5 per cent in 1912, 'largely through the efforts of the 'Plunket Society', a health society established by Lord and Lady Plunket.[13]

Like the WNHA, the St Ultan's staff was concerned about the health of the mother and infant since both were connected. Infant and maternal mortality was silent mortality. Deaths associated with political difficulties were commented on, yet the quieter tragedy of infant death continued unabated. Between 1911 and 1915 the infant mortality rate was 91 per 1,000; hence for every 100 infants, nine did not see their first birthday. Dublin had one of the worse records for infant mortality. In 1915, the rate for Dublin County Borough was 160 per 1,000. Not surprisingly, there were dramatic class differences. The mortality rate for children under five years for the professional class was 7 per 1,000 of the total population; this rose to 22 for the middle class, and a staggering

120 for the offspring of those described as hawkers, porters and labourers.[14] Given the dire state of housing for the Dublin poor, these figures should not surprise us. Charles Cameron spent more than thirty years as Chief Medical Officer for Dublin. In 1913 he noted that one-third of families lived in single rooms and in the 'homes of the very poor the seeds of infective disease are nursed as it were in a hothouse.'[15]

Furthermore, urban areas were generally far more dangerous for infants than rural areas. The infant mortality rate was twice as high in urban areas.[16] Lynn resolved to stem the growth of these deadly seeds and improve the grim infant mortality statistics through a variety of measures.

ST ULTAN'S

St Ultan's Hospital for Infants, or Teach Ultáin, was established in May, 1919 by Lynn and ffrench-Mullen in response to medico-social conditions in Dublin. It was not unusual for women to establish hospitals. In the nineteenth century, female religious orders had established hospitals such as St Vincent's (1834) and the Mater (1861) in Dublin. These institutions facilitated the development of the nursing profession, but they rarely provided opportunities for female doctors. However, women in Britain, and elsewhere, founded institutions in the late- nineteenth century to facilitate women's access to the medical profession. These provided employment opportunities for female professionals.[17] International developments also motivated Lynn and ffrench-Mullen, as they noted that Dundee, Manchester and London had opened hospitals for women and children.[18] St Ultan's was unique in Ireland as it was the only hospital that was entirely managed by women. Males were employed for specialities, but the hospital had a positive discrimination policy and favoured female staff. This may have been motivated by Lynn's experience of professional prejudice. By the 1920s, women constituted 11 per cent of the medical profession but they were deprived of professional opportunities enjoyed by male physicians.[19] Hence, St Ultan's was established for both political and professional reasons. Lynn and her republican friends were all too aware of the needs of the Dublin poor but they were also providing a niche for female doctors in St Ultan's.

As noted earlier, the female members of Sinn Féin who had established Cumann na dTeachtaire (League of Women Delegates) were concerned about child welfare. The British Ministry of Health noted that there was a large increase in attendance at venereal disease clinics in 1919. Outpatient attendance at the VD clinics in England and Wales doubled; from 488,137 in 1918 to 1,002,791 in 1919. This may have been due, in part, to greater public awareness. In 1917, there was 'a sudden rise in infant mortality attributed to syphilis in the death returns; the rise being greater proportionately amongst illegitimate than legitimate infants'. In Ireland, the Lock Hospital (which was specifically for female venereal disease patients) noted that attendance at the outpatient department was 900 for the year 1920–21; this was 'an increase of upwards of 600 upon the previous year'. The extern department had only been introduced in 1919. By 1922–23, the numbers being treated declined. The annual report referred to 23 'healthy children' who were born to mothers infected with the disease.[20]

The inspiration for the name of the hospital came from Lynn who toured County Meath. Ultan, a seventh-century Bishop of Ardbraccan, near Navan, looked after the children of Meath, during a yellow plague.[21] He was a role model for the hospital. Lynn was particularly impressed by the rich archaeological remains in the County. In August 1919, ffrench-Mullen and Lynn spent a 'glorious day at Slane, pilgrimage to Holy Well'. Later they visited the prehistoric burial sites at Newgrange and Dowth.[22]

ST ULTAN'S STAFF

Many of the women associated with St Ultan's in its earliest years shared the political outlook and professional interests of Lynn. Their medical concerns for women and children, as well as their political experiences, mirror the kind of activism that St Ultan's nurtured.

Dr Katherine Maguire was known to Lynn through suffrage activity and both were interested in social medicine. In 1898, Maguire's paper to the Alexandra College Guild on 'Social

Conditions of the Dublin Poor', motivated the guild to establish model tenement houses. Maguire had a private practice in Merrion Square in Dublin. She also opened a Free Dispensary at Harold's Cross. As part of her interest in alleviating the causes of ill health, she bought four tenement houses in Tyrone Street and let them at a minimum rent. As a lecturer on hygiene at Alexandra College (her lectures on health began in 1893), she was described as an 'exceptionally gifted teacher'. Although a member of the Academy of Medicine, according to Lynn, Maguire's 'self-effacing disposition did not permit her to speak or to show cases' at the Academy. Enthusiastic about women's rights, she was described by Lynn, somewhat oxymoronically, as a 'non-militant suffragette'.[23]

Corkonian Alice Barry (1880–1955) had received her licence to practise medicine in 1904. She was associated with the Women's National Health Association from its beginning in 1907. However, there was a eugenic strain to some of the WNHA's pronouncements. Furthermore, Dr Marion Andrews, who was associated with the work of the WNHA, was also honorary secretary of the Belfast Eugenics Society.[24] Ironically, Barry, who did not share Aberdeen's eugenic views, was to prevent the expansion of St Ultan's because she was reluctant to counter the Catholic Archbishop's insinuations in the 1930s regarding alleged eugenic practices in St Ultan's. Barry was in charge of the nine Dublin Babies' Clubs, which had been established by the WNHA between 1912 and 1929. She had also worked as a medical officer in Kilbrittain, West Cork and shared Lynn's nationalism. Appointed as resident medical superintendent of the WNHA's Peamount Sanatorium in 1929, her interest in tuberculosis eradication was evident in her membership of the Irish National Anti-Tuberculosis League. Like Lynn, she made her home available to republicans during the War of Independence. As visiting physician to St Ultan's and a member of the medical and general committee she was influential and ultimately divisive.[25]

Elizabeth Tennant also worked with Lynn in St Ultan's for many years. She received her licentiate from the Royal College of Physicians and Surgeons in 1894, and practised in Harrington Street, Dublin, between 1894 and 1937. As an honorary visiting physician to St Ultan's, she was a 'valued member' of staff as well as medical officer to St Catherine's School and Orphanage in Dublin. Her large general practice in Dublin specialised in midwifery. A hagiographical obituary suggested 'her devotion to her work and to the hospital is acknowledged by all those connected with it to have been one of the biggest factors in the success of the institution'.[26]

Ella Webb (Ovenden) was the daughter of the Dean of St Patrick's Cathedral, hence she shared Lynn's Church of Ireland background.[27] Furthermore, like Lynn, she was educated at Alexandra College, and she also studied at Queen's College, Harley Street, London and at Göttingen, in Germany. Although Webb wanted to study medicine, she first graduated with a natural science degree from the RUI. In 1904, she graduated with first place in her medical degree from Cecilia Street to the delight of 'Speranza' from *St Stephen's*. The Catholic University Magazine triumphantly announced that it 'was a record to gain it over the heads of so many competitors of the sterner sex, which, until recent years, regarded medicine as exclusively its own ground'.[28] Webb was awarded her Master's in Medicine in 1906. Like Dr Maguire, she won the prestigious travelling scholarship and studied in Vienna. After marriage to George Webb, a Fellow of TCD, she combined family commitments with private practice and a free evening dispensary in Kevin Street. Her busy professional life also included work as a demonstrator of physiology in the Women's Department of the TCD Medical School, as well as election to the visiting staff of the Adelaide Hospital, as assistant physician to the children's department. She was also prominent in the WNHA. In 1918, Webb was appointed as anaesthetist to the Adelaide.

Her work at St Ultan's reinforced her interest in paediatrics. Webb founded the Stillorgan Children's Sunshine Home. In 1924, she had written a paper on 'Sunshine and Health' for the Alexandra Guild Conference. This interest coincided with her research on rickets. Subsequently, a committee of women 'interested in child welfare had been formed to provide an open-air convalescent home'. Ultimately, this led to the development of the Sunshine Home, which provided much-needed holiday homes for deprived inner city children.[29]

Webb's work with Lynn and Dorothy Stopford Price in St Ultan's further enhanced the reputation of female doctors in the prevention of diseases, particularly those which were exacerbated by socio-economic deprivation.[30] Barry, Lynn and Webb, through their work in St Ultan's and elsewhere, personified the link between nineteenth-century philanthropy and twentieth-century professionalism.

Nan Dougan was the first matron at St Ultan's. Lynn may have known her from Sir Patrick Dun's where they both worked. Dougan had worked in a children's hospital in Manchester and was a central figure in St Ultan's for more than twenty years. Dougan's 'right-hand woman' was Miss Mulligan who came for a postgraduate course in 1923 and stayed for twenty-six years.[31] The first chairman of St Ultan's was Lucy Griffin, an inspector of children for the Rathdown Union in south Dublin. However, probably the most important members of staff in St Ultan's were the nurses. They spent the most time in the hospital. Lynn always employed a maid who ensured that she did not have to worry about domestic issues. 'Jane good to me', Lynn admitted in March 1921.[32] Likewise, the silent service provided by the nurses was vital for the survival of St Ultan's.[33]

ESTABLISHMENT

These vigorous and strong-minded women were determined that St Ultan's would make its mark in the Dublin medical world and provide much-needed medical facilities. Not surprisingly, politics played a role in its development. In May 1918, at the first meeting which was to lead to the establishment of the hospital, Lynn, who read a paper on venereal disease, declared her desire to educate the public on VD. Barry proposed, and Lucy Griffin seconded the motion that 'This conference of Irishwomen note with appreciation that the corporations of Dublin and Belfast have taken up the question of venereal disease, and urge those bodies to see that every soldier who lands at Irish ports is guaranteed free from disease.'[34]

The St Ultan's founders, and Lynn in particular, were part of a group known as Sláinte na nGaedheal which was interested in the health of the nation. They were part of a national movement which sought the cultural, moral, physical and intellectual regeneration of the Irish people through organisations such as the Gaelic League and the Gaelic Athletic Association (GAA). The committee feared for the health of the nation's children. The St Ultan's committee recommended that 'local authorities under the Children's Act . . . [should] have such infants [suffering from syphilis] immediately removed for treatment to hospitals on diagnosis of their disease by the medical officer of the district, and that copies of this resolution be sent to Boards of Guardians and local authorities'. They also asked whether there was provision for syphilitic infants in any hospital.[35] By May, the committee had sent Lucy Griffin to see P.T. Daly, a nationalist member of Dublin Corporation, regarding health facilities. These early issues underline a number of different developments which affected Lynn and her colleagues. The increasing role of the state (including local government) in medicine, and the growing importance of paediatrics and public health (the two were closely linked), provided a focus for Lynn to express her political beliefs and professional concerns.

By July 1918, arrangements were being made to buy 37 Charlemont Street, the eventual site of the hospital. When the influenza epidemic reached Dublin in November 1918, the committee appealed directly to the public. Lynn and ffrench-Mullen met Dr William Walsh, the Roman Catholic Archbishop. It was reported in the minutes that 'the Archbishop never likes [the words 'would not' were scored out] to share in the starting of an enterprise like this for which he is not directly responsible, [and] that he will be guided in his support by the advice of his medical advisers. [He also] recognises the need of such a hospital . . . [and] he is sympathetic towards it'. The committee published the Archbishop's approval in the daily papers on 1 January 1919. It is revealing that they thought it advisable to gain the support of the Roman Catholic Archbishop. Furthermore, Walsh was a staunch nationalist and would have known Lynn through her work on the Sinn Féin Public Health Committee. There is no mention of a meeting with his Church of Ireland counterpart, though Lynn was a member of the Church of Ireland. The hospital opened on Ascension Thursday, the 29 May 1919. 'May the Lord bless our work', Lynn wrote.[36]

A book entitled *Leabhar Ultáin: The Book of Saint Ultan* was compiled in 1920 by Katherine MacCormack and sold to support the hospital. It contained an introduction by the historian Alice Stopford Green (the aunt of Dr Dorothy Stopford Price), poems, drawings and pictures by George Russell, Maud Gonne MacBride, Thomas Bodkin, Harry Clarke and Jack B. Yeats among others. This enterprise proved to be financially rewarding as the book made more than £90.[37] In this way, Lynn and her friends used cultural nationalists to promote their hospital.

Every year, St Ultan's organised a pilgrimage-cum-picnic to Ardbraccan, the site of St Ultan's well and his tiny church on the saint's feast day in September. This bilingual and multi-denominational outing usually consisted of a rosary and evensong in Irish. Lynn wanted to Gaelicise the Church of Ireland liturgy, and she was taking Irish classes in Dublin in the 1910s.[38] In 1921 the committee thanked de Valera for permitting them to advertise that 'he was coming to the Derideacht' (outing), as it increased attendance five-fold. These outings were greatly enjoyed by Lynn and her friends, providing the rain stayed away. In 1923, a special train to Navan was organised, and after a feis at Ardbraccan, there were competitions in music, singing, lilting, whistling, dancing and skipping, as well as prizes for the best exhibit of wild flowers.[39] These activities reflect Lynn's love of nature and Irish traditions.

Financing the hospital was the biggest challenge. The 'amusements committee' of St Ultan's played a major role in keeping the auditors content. Given the general poverty in Ireland, not to mention the fact that Ireland was teetering on the edge of the War of Independence, and the limited funds for public health, Lynn used all connections to support the hospital. The hospital organised céilís and fêtes, one of which was held in St Enda's, the all-Irish school established by Pearse.[40] The Navan Excursion Committee, which organised the trip to Ardbraccan, gave a cheque for £285 to the hospital. Lynn's friendship with Sr Columba, the Reverend Mother at St Michael's, the Loreto Convent in Navan, ensured support from that quarter. They 'sent a large consignment of woollies made after the hospital pattern for the Babies'.[41] In the same year, 1921, funds from the United States, facilitated the work of the hospital when the Women's Education League of San Francisco sent $32.[42] Clearly, the promotion work undertaken by St Ultan's staff, particularly ffrench-Mullen, the hospital's administrator, was reaping rewards. Classical concerts, with ffrench-Mullen's brother Douglas and her sister Eileen as musicians, took place on Thursdays, between November and April, 1920–21, despite the War of Independence.[43]

Lynn used her republican political links to fund the hospital. The White Cross, which was established to support republican families, gave £2,000 to St Ultan's in 1927. This was used to develop an outpatients department, which was opened by Alice Stopford Green in 1928. It included modern equipment from the United States.[44] Lynn loved the most up-to-date inventions. For example, she introduced the Abt's electric breast pump, which helped mothers to produce milk.[45] Lynn was a particularly strong advocate of breastfeeding and she wrote in the periodical, *Old Ireland*, that 'nature made no mistake when she designed that mammals should suckle their young'.[46] The link between reducing infant mortality and breastfeeding was still being promoted in South America and the Caribbean in the twenty-first century.[47]

ACTIVITIES

The events associated with St Ultan's clearly reflect Lynn's cultural republicanism. Many of the hospital's activities were advertised in Irish thus linking them with nationalist movements. The hospital maintained its connections with individuals associated with Irish nationalists. Not all of the hospital supporters were nationalists, however. Lady Carson, the wife of the unionist leader, Edward Carson, donated a goat who was promptly named Carson. However, the goats, which were essential in providing tuberculosis-free milk for the patients, waged war on the Matron and the gardener, and were sent elsewhere.[48] An anonymous donor in San Francisco gave £25 for a cot to be named after Rory O'Connor, an executed republican. Only St Ultan's would have a goat called Carson and a cot named Rory O'Connor![49]

St Ultan's concern for the health of mothers extended to running a holiday home for them in Baldoyle. One of the aims of the hospital was to be 'a university for mothers'. In 1917, Edward Coey Bigger, the Medical Commissioner of the Local Government Board for Ireland, declared that Irish women were 'not fitted for motherhood'. The 'great evil is lack of good mother-craft', he surmised.[50] Lynn and her colleagues agreed with this assessment. The staff strongly encouraged mothers to attend lectures at the hospital. Welfare workers also attended; the hospital declared that one of their main aims was 'to spread knowledge'.[51] They were therefore part of an international movement to train mothers. Dr Newman, the Chief Medical Officer to the Board of Education in England, pointed out that infant mortality was due to the 'ignorance of the mother and the remedy is the education of the mother'.[52] Educating women was a particular interest of Lynn's, and St Ultan's provided her the opportunity to spread the gospel of cleanliness. This focus on education reflects the middle-class bias of Lynn and her colleagues. It was they who would instruct mothers. In her work on tuberculosis in Belfast, Isabel Magill suggested that 'hygiene which concentrated upon moral and domestic reform was seen as part of the process by which the poor were to be subdued, modified, improved and moulded into a cogent economic force'.[53] On occasion, this focus on education could dampen the social radicalism of St Ultan's. Without the political will at a national level to improve the living conditions of patients and their parents, then the infant mortality rate could not be radically reduced. The need for the hospital was obvious given that in their first year, of the 53 infants treated, 23 died, a shocking mortality rate. It is worth noting that in 1925 'more than half (281) the total number of deaths of illegitimate infants occurred in Dublin county and city'. These infants were six times more likely than their legitimate contemporaries to die before the age of one.[54] Given the high number of illegitimate infants at the hospital, the high mortality rate is tragic but not unexpected. Given the presence of death and Lynn's religious outlook, the tiny mortuary contained a prie-Dieu and 'a picture of Christ with a dead babe in his arms'. Appropriately, the site of the hospital was described as being on Charlemont Bridge, 'the boundary line between prosperity and adversity'. St Ultan's followed 'the initiative and lines of the "Manchester Baby Hospital"'.[55] Despite her political distrust of Britain, Lynn was happy to learn from British medical developments, and Dr Catherine Chisholm of the Manchester Infant

Hospital gave a lecture in the Royal College of Surgeons in May 1920, as part of St Ultan's Week.[56]

Nonetheless, Lynn did not lose sight of her political agenda and cleverly merged national and medical aspirations. When Pearse's play, *The Singer*, was being performed at the Abbey Theatre for St Ultan's, Lynn gave a speech which emphasised that infant mortality 'was in direct proportion to the amount of money that the parents had, and it was the duty of every man and woman who had money enough for simple necessities of life and something over to give that surplus to assist children who, without their aid, must inevitably perish'.[57] In 1922 ffrench-Mullen wrote to a newspaper that the hospital had 'no association, direct or indirect, with any political party or organisation. Any person making statements to the contrary will be proceeded against.'[58] Evidently, some were wary of the hospital because of the political prominence of some of its staff. Lynn, however, was undaunted and she maintained Irish-American connections to further her Ultan's vision. In a letter to Mrs Mary McWhorter, President of the Celtic Cross Association of Chicago, she thanked her for the 'generous donation for St Ultan's. It is indeed a God-send, and we hope many a little baby who would otherwise have perished, will live and thrive through the kindness of our good friends in Chicago'. More revealingly, she wrote, 'I shall always remember that evening in Mountjoy Square when I met you and Terence MacSwiney'.[59] The latter's significant involvement in the republican movement and his subsequent death after a lengthy hunger strike galvanised nationalists. Clearly, Lynn saw her St Ultan's work as part of national regeneration and was not willing to shed her republican credentials. On the contrary, she used them to promote the hospital. However, given her wide-ranging political activities, particularly her involvement in republican support groups, St Ultan's was seen as a threat to the Irish Free State. While Lynn was in Paris and Geneva in December 1922 with Áine Ceannt in the hope that the hospital was raided. (They would extract money from the International Red Cross on behalf of republicans.) While no incriminating material was found, Lynn's letters to ffrench-Mullen were confiscated. Lynn described the Irish Free State as a 'farce'. While there was no love lost between Lynn and the Free Staters, her devotion to ffrench-Mullen was obvious. 'I do praise my K.L. for resting & I am so glad Emer [Helena Molony] was with you.' Lynn ended her letter with, 'my own love to you, my own K.L. I send you the only thing we got for nothing so far 10,000,000 kisses K.L.'[60] It should not surprise us that St Ultan's was searched when Lynn was out of the country. The irony is that the raiders only captured affectionate letters between two female republicans. These letters would lie undisturbed for many years in military archives.

Lynn was careful, despite her willingness to appear in most photographs of St Ultan's, not to garner all the credit for the hospital. According to one newspaper she praised her 'able and willing' colleagues, without whose help the hospital would not exist. 'They had, all of them, practical knowledge of the situation, they were workers amongst the children.'[61] Furthermore, they were proud of the fact that they were doing 'good by stealth', though they would meet control by stealth when they tried to expand their activities in the 1930s.[62]

DEVELOPMENT

The major challenge facing St Ultan's was reducing its horrendous mortality rate. The biggest killer of infants in the 1920s was gastroenteritis, a highly infectious disease. Because many of the patients had this disease the risk of infecting others was high. The National Children's Hospital (Harcourt Street) did not accept children with infectious diseases. Though they were a hospital for 'poor children', like St Ultan's, their mortality rate was significantly lower. In 1928 they admitted 271 patients, and 36 died in the hospital.[63] In order to understand the difficulties facing infants with infectious diseases, St Ultan's had opened a new bacteriological and pathological laboratory with the Celtic Cross Association of Chicago funds.[64] In 1926 Dr Margaret Enright was appointed bacteriologist. She was a first-class honours medical graduate and had been an assistant bacteriologist at UCC. She conducted research on the microbes found on babies' comforters. Lynn was very aware of the effect of environment on the health of children. Just prior to the establishment of the hospital she noted in her diary, 'poor little Flinter baby died in mg, just after we had been there. It had no chance in that filthy place.' By the late 1920s, St Ultan's had thirty-five cots, a matron, a sister, five staff nurses, and six probationers. Patients came from all over the country. In keeping with the social outlook of the hospital, annual reports contain detailed records of the background of the patients, including the proportion whose fathers were unemployed. In 1924 this was 44 per cent. The report also noted that 15 per cent of the patients were 'illegitimate'. Nationally, in 1926, the infant mortality rates compared favourably with Northern Ireland and unfavourably with Britain:

74 per 1,000
Irish Free State

112 per 1,000
Belfast

118 per 1,000
Derry

64 per 1,000
London

80 per 1,000
Edinburgh.

Revealingly, the infant mortality rate was a staggering 30 per cent in 1928 for illegitimate children.[65] St Ultan's was obviously providing a service for those who badly needed it, but they were unable to prevent mortality in most cases. In October 1922, it was proposed by Dr Elizabeth Tennant and seconded by Dr Alice Barry that 'cases of infant girls should not be admitted while there are cases of vaginal discharge in the house – subsequently girl infants admitted should be kept under observation for a time before being admitted to the ordinary wards. All cases of vaginal discharge now in the hospital should be discharged as soon as possible.'[66] The following January, when Lynn was not at the medical committee meeting, it was decided that the infants with vaginal discharge should not be treated in the hospital and 'the child with no parents can be sent to the Lock Hospital'.[67] The hospital had evidently moved considerably from its original concern with VD. Now there was nothing facing a syphilitic infant except the Lock Hospital. There were great concerns about the socio-economic conditions of families. While little could be done about a child infected with VD, there was a sense that improved medical care might alleviate distress. In 1926 it was suggested that an antenatal clinic might be established. Like the Babies' Clubs they sought to give advice to expectant mothers and, crucially, given the poverty of so many families, to provide meals or supplement the home diet with milk and eggs, and give clothing, 'where necessary'. The medical committee also planned to have a consulting gynaecologist and a trained nurse at the clinic. However, these great plans would come to nothing without funds.[68]

St Ultan's also sought to support families through the provision of improved housing. In the 1930s the St Ultan's Hospital Utility Society was to establish model tenement homes in order to break the cycle of poverty and illhealth.[69] This was not an unusual development as the impoverished Irish state had encouraged the establishment of utility societies in order to facilitate the growth of housing.[70] However, while the St Ultan's flats were eventually built in the 1940s, and named the ffrench-Mullen flats, the management of the flats was given over to Dublin Corporation. Difficulties with collecting rents and with legal representatives provoked the general committee of the hospital to hand over the flats to the corporation.[71] While the St Ultan's staff may have been seen as a 'little panzer division',[72] there was little they could do with reluctant tenants. Nonetheless, it was an admirable effort to establish model homes which were still in use in 2002.

Alongside her interest in better homes, Lynn preached the virtues of cleanliness and fresh air. She was heavily involved with An Óige (a youth organisation) and her cottage at Glenmalure in County Wicklow was given to them after her death. In 1928, she gave a talk on breastfeeding where she pointed out that 'breast milk is the baby's birthright'. It was 'nourishment provided by God'. She also encouraged her less-than-convinced patients to enjoy the 'bracing effect' of fresh air.[73] These ideas were current elsewhere. During the 1920s in England, classes in 'mothercraft' were organised and, according to Jane Lewis, a series of rhymes helped drive the points home:

> Baby thrives at Mother's breast
> That's the food he likes best
> Give when his meal hour strikes
> Not at any time he likes
> ... If healthy children you would raise
> Open windows nights and days.[74]

Despite her political commitments Lynn still found time to attend medical lectures.[75] However, most people were occupied by the upheavals of the War of Independence and the Civil War.

INTERNATIONAL AFFAIRS

Throughout the 1920s, Lynn visited the Continent and Britain on her holidays, but she always managed to visit hospitals during her sojourns abroad. Prior to her departure for the United States in October 1925, St Ultan's welcomed a group of physicians from the United States and Canada who were part of the Inter-State Post-Graduate Assembly. St Ultan's demonstrated 'its methods of treatment'.[76] Two months later, a 'U.S.A. Dr Kerley' visited the hospital and was 'much interested in all he saw'.[77] Dr Kerley facilitated Lynn in the United States by writing letters of introduction. Lynn clearly wanted to maintain her international contacts and may have known some of these physicians from her postgraduate work in the United States. The Rockefeller Foundation was very active in promoting public health initiatives. Lynn contacted Dr Matthew Russell of the Rockefeller Foundation on 3 November 1925. She emphasised that 'Miss ffrench-Mullen and I would be very grateful' for an interview. Their aspiration was that Dr Russell would introduce them to medical practitioners. Furthermore, they were 'most anxious' to obtain his 'guidance and advice as to our program here, having come to make a survey of Child Welfare and Preventive Medicine in your progressive Country'.[78] Furthermore, she used Irish – American links to support St Ultan's. These links were enhanced during her two-month visit to the United States in 1925, where she met a score of US physicians including those who had established infant hospitals in the United States, such as Dr Hess who had established a Preventorium in New York. She was particularly impressed by the Mount Sinai Hospital in New York and marvelled at the wonderful facilities of US hospitals. While in Boston, Lynn met the paediatrician, William Emerson, whose book *Nutrition and Growth in Children* was published in 1922.[79] He gave her 'much literature' and said that doctors 'only treat disease'. His views on prevention would have chimed with Lynn's. Furthermore, Lynn and ffrench-Mullen had an office on Fifth Avenue, New York for the St Ultan's Fund.[80] Not surprisingly, given Lynn's awareness of socio-medical developments, she met the well known paediatrician, Dr Josephine Baker, whom she described as 'a wonderful worker'. Lynn 'learnt much' from Baker. Perhaps she was a role model for Lynn, since Baker was 'an acknowledged pioneer in the field of child health' and set up the first Child Health Bureau in 1908. Two years later she organised Little Mothers' Clubs so that older girls would know how to look after their younger siblings. Baker was most associated with the Children's Bureau which gave advice on child health to American mothers, and it has been compared with the Babies' Clubs in Ireland.[81]

Lynn and ffrench-Mullen's activities were advertised on their return. *The Irish Independent* noted that they 'organised a small drive for funds, and also made a survey of baby hospitals and child welfare generally'.[82] According to the St Ultan's Annual Report for 1927, Lynn and ffrench-Mullen collected $909 in the US.[83] American republican connections also proved to be generous as the hospital benefited from 'Irish Republican Bond Certificate Holders'.[84]

NATURE AND SPIRITUALITY

How did Lynn maintain her motivation and commitment? Throughout the difficult years of the early 1920s Lynn's serenity was sustained by religion and nature. At the height of the War of

Independence, she travelled to Kilbride in County Meath for Sunday service. Afterwards, she picked 'cowslips on hill. Birds and quietness so refreshing.'[85] She needed these distractions given that her home was raided and she frequently railed at the level of violence perpetrated by the British Army and the Black and Tans. People were 'terrorised' by them, she wrote. Characteristically, she sought succour from her faith: 'Thou O God art our Defence.'[86] One can also see Lynn taking solace from history. Her diaries are organised so that she can reflect on the previous years. In April 1921 she wrote, 'It was very much like this day 5 yrs. Thought much of Sean Connolly.'[87] For Lynn nationalism and spirituality were often intertwined. On St Patrick's Day, 1925 she wrote, 'S. Patrick's, the joy of a Gaelic Celebration!' Lynn regularly attended a service in Irish at St Andrew's and greatly enjoyed it.[88]

Her family and friends also sustained her. Relations with her father had improved. In December 1920, Lynn received a letter to say she could go home at Christmas, if she did not 'have demonstration' or 'see people who are not their visitors'. She complied with her family's requests and returned home 'joyfully'. It was 'lovely to be home'. It was her first Christmas in Cong for four years. However, her father's sermon on St Stephen's Day 'annoyed' her. 'He should say nothing if he can only think of police.'[89] Her father sided with the authorities. Ironically, she suggested that her family 'only see one side.'[90] Clearly her inflexibility and partisanship was not unique. Lynn's father died on 8 April 1923. Though they had had their political differences, her grief at his passing was all too evident. Her friend Áine (Fanny) Ceannt wrote that Lynn was 'terribly cut up' when he died.[91] 'We were glad when he was at rest, now we can grieve for him', Lynn wrote.[92] Though she had been estranged from her father during the Rising, she had made her peace with him before his death. In February 1919 she mentioned dining with him; she was 'glad to see him . . . looking very well.'[93] Later in the year, her sister Nan told her that 'they would like me at home, only no one must know I am there.'[94] According to Dr Dónal Caird, Lynn described her father as 'the best person she had known in her life'.[95] The family, however, was less than united. John, her brother, was not at his father's funeral, and later in the year, she asked, 'Where is he to-day?'[96] He had married and left his wife and three children in Australia while he went to New York. Lynn was in occasional contact with his family, since she received a letter in March 1923 from his wife Anna, but the family had had not 'written for years'.[97] John returned to Ireland in May 1926, much to Lynn's joy. He was to stay with her before going to the United States.[98] Lynn obviously saw herself as responsible for her siblings after her father's death. With the ill health of her older sister, Nan, and Muriel's decision to live in Northern Ireland, this placed the onus on Lynn to keep a careful eye on her wayward brother.[99] She also looked after her elderly Aunt Florence and usually celebrated Christmas with her. (Ffrench-Mullen performed the same role for her brother Douglas, who seemed to be a model of inconsistency.) The most important person in Lynn's life was her great friend Madeleine. In December 1926, she wrote 'we are living together nearly 11 years now D.G.'[100] They shared the same ideological outlook and sustained each other through the trials of the 1910s and '20s.

Of course, Lynn's work was also made possible by the maids she employed at her home. On occasion, she seemed harsh. Jane, who had worked for Lynn from at least 1916, was given notice in 1924. Lynn simply wrote, 'she is too long here'.[101] However, it is possible that she then went on to work for Muriel in County Down. Lynn's active life was facilitated by the silent help of Ireland's Janes; a quiet army of nurses worked in St Ultan's. For Lynn and her colleagues, the nature of the new Irish state did not permit major socio-economic change. Hence their work would always be a drop in the ocean of Dublin's poverty.

CONCLUSION

In 1932 Nora Connolly O'Brien suggested that 'it is regrettable that Irishwomen should have the ability to return to the everyday task, that having won the right to share in the dangers of war, they should have relinquished their right to share in the dangers of peace'.[102] Lynn and others had endured the dangers of the War of Independence and Civil War, but then they endured the frustration of discriminatory legislation, such as the Juries Act of 1927. W.T.

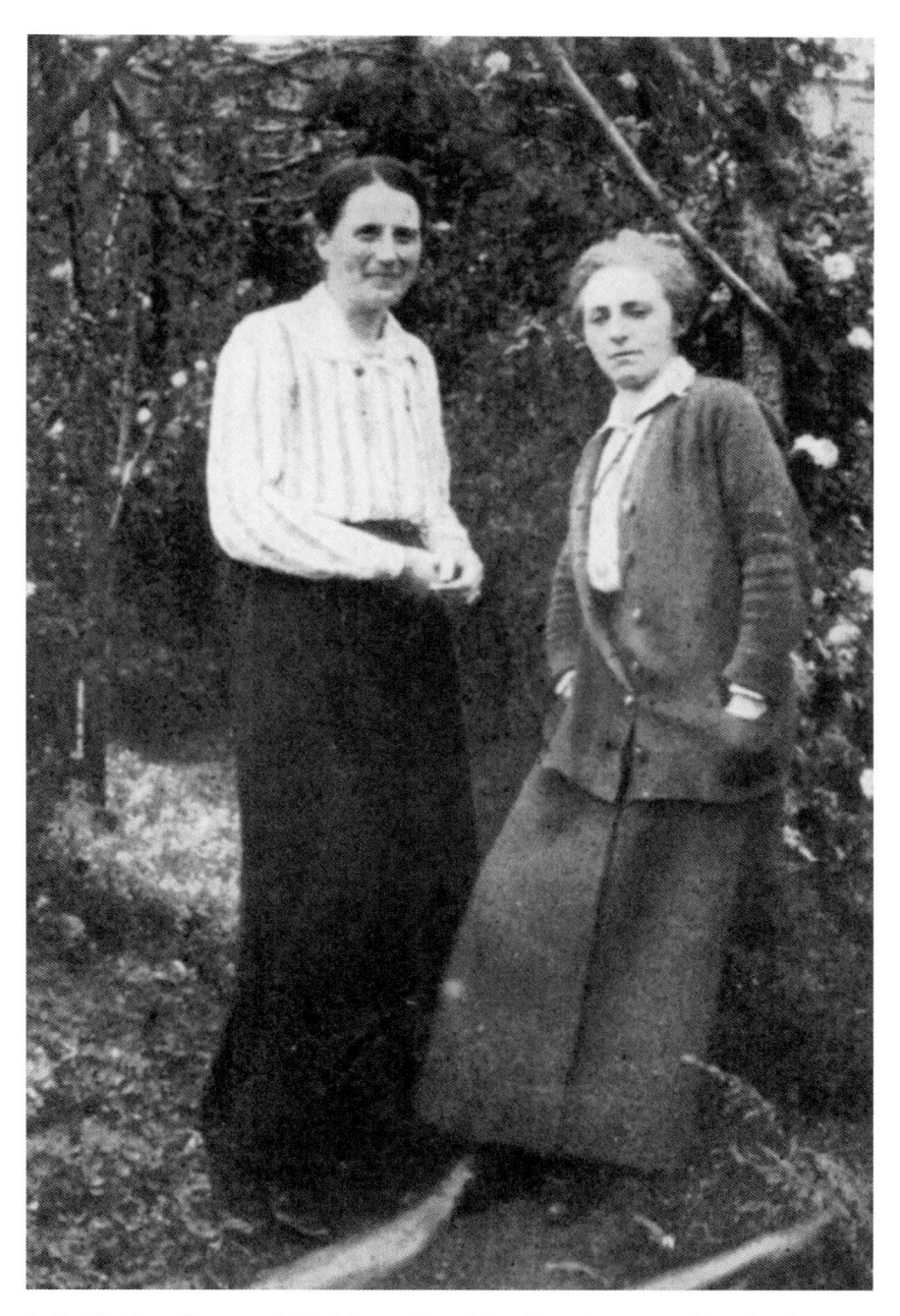

1. Dr Kathleen Lynn and Madeleine ffrench-Mullen, *circa*, 1919. (*St. Ultan's Annual Report, 1945,* Courtesy of the Royal College of Physicians of Ireland).

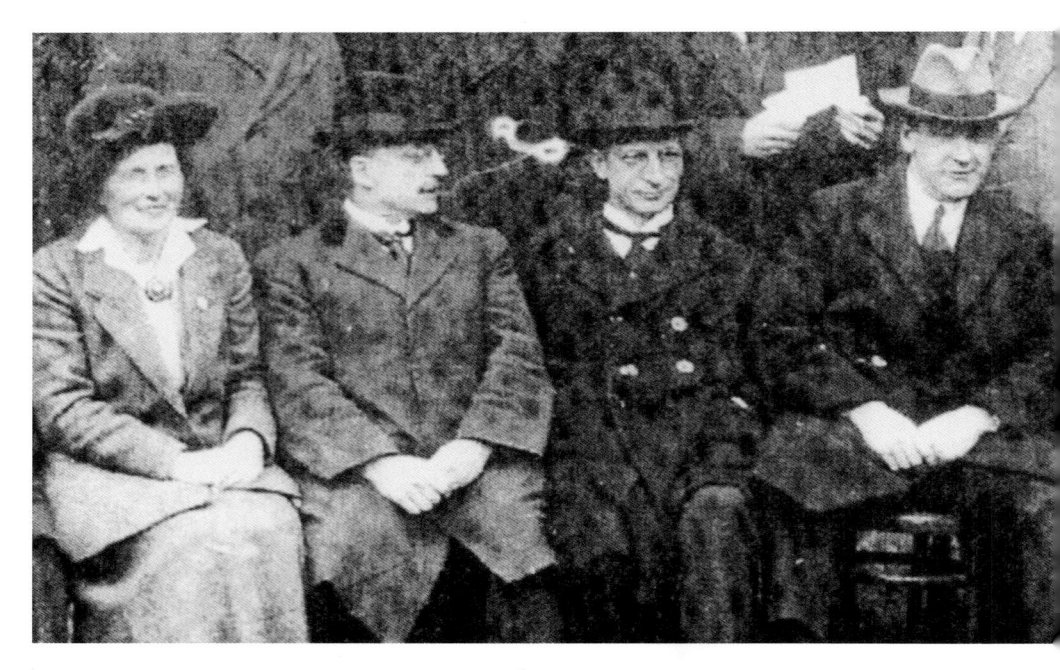

2. Dr. Kathleen Lynn, Arthur Griffith, Éamon de Valera and Michael Collins, 1921. (Courtesy of the Royal College of Physicians of Ireland).

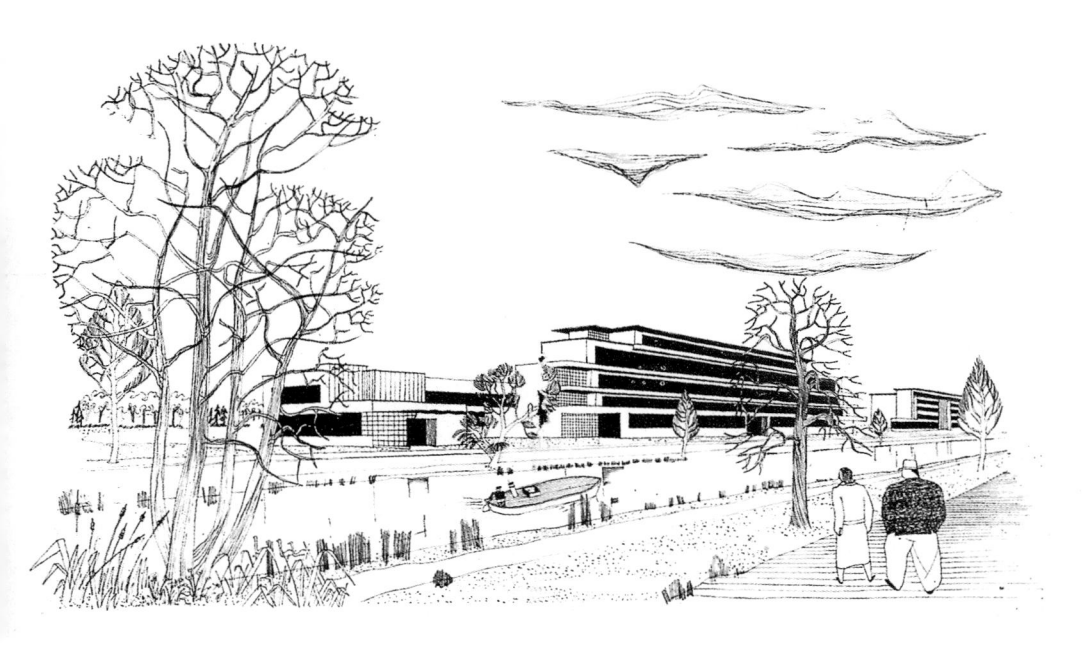

3. Dream Hospital, what St. Ultan's might have been, *circa* 1936. (*St. Ultan's Annual Report, 1945,* Courtesy of the Royal College of Physicians of Ireland).

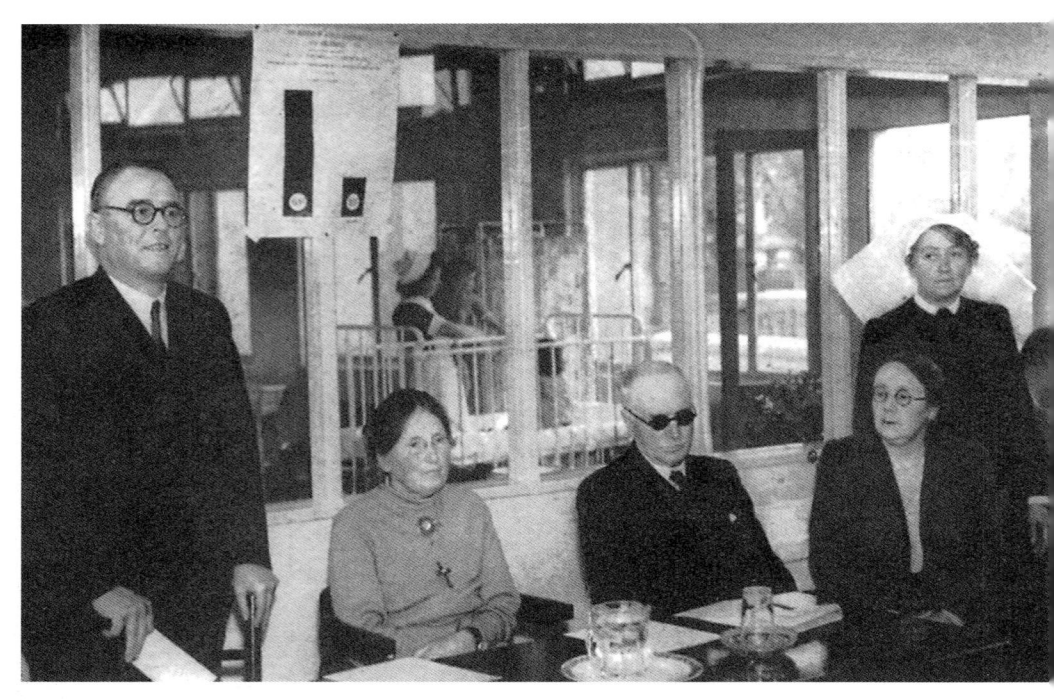

4. St. Ultan's Annual General Meeting, 1944, Dr. Kathleen Lynn, Dr. Thomas Gillman Moorhead, Dr. Dorothy Stopford Price and Sister Mulligan, the Matron). (*St. Ultan's Annual Report, 1945*, Courtesy of the Royal College of Physicians of Ireland).

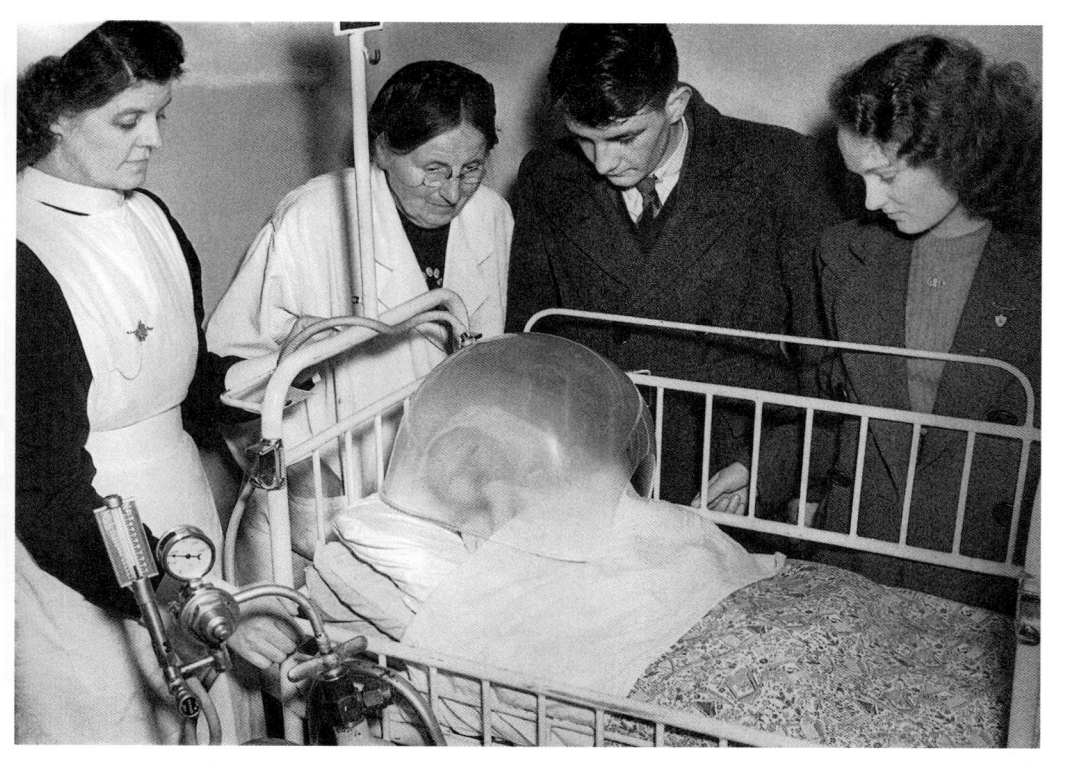

5. Dr. Kathleen Lynn and St. Ultan's patient with Oxygen Hood, with Rathmines Junior Red Cross and a nurse, 1948. (Courtesy of the Royal College of Physicians of Ireland).

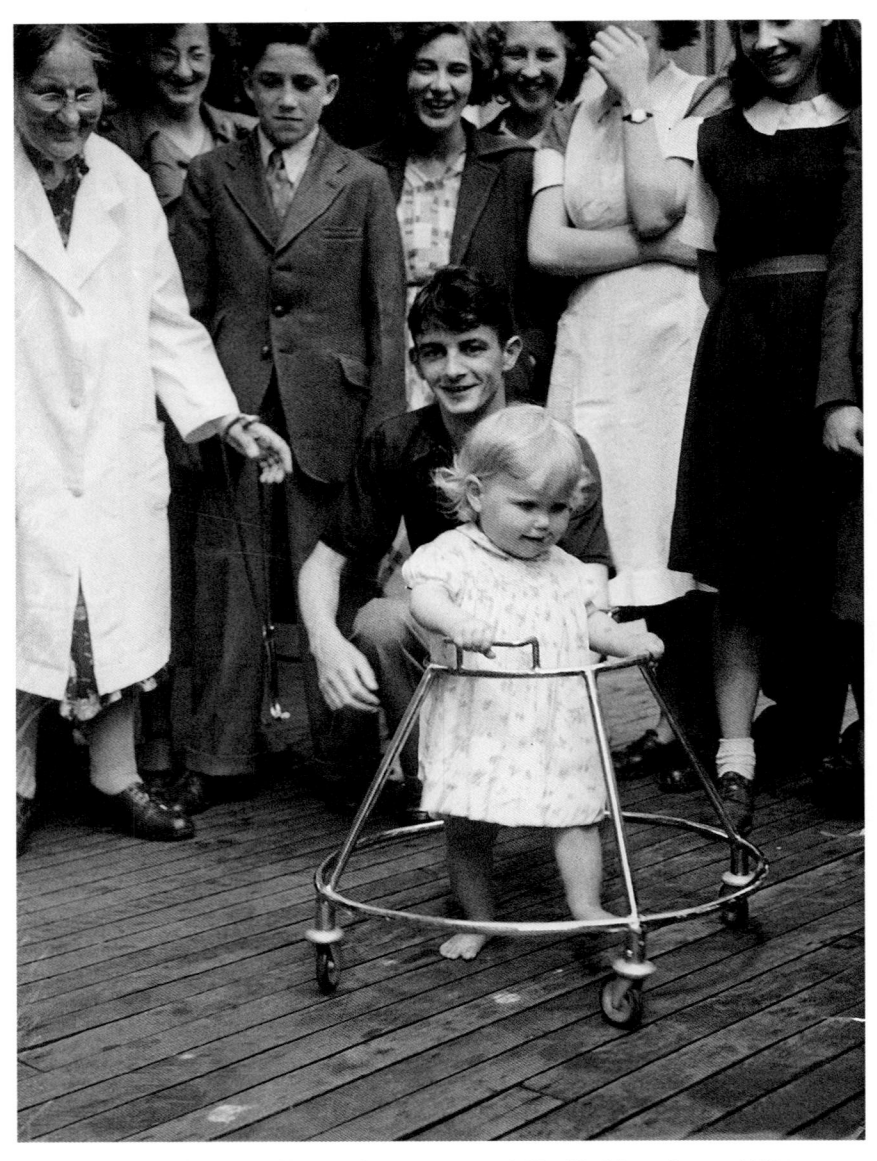

6. Child on stroller, possibly a polio victim, with Dr. Kathleen Lynn, 1950. (Courtesy of the Royal College of Physicians of Ireland).

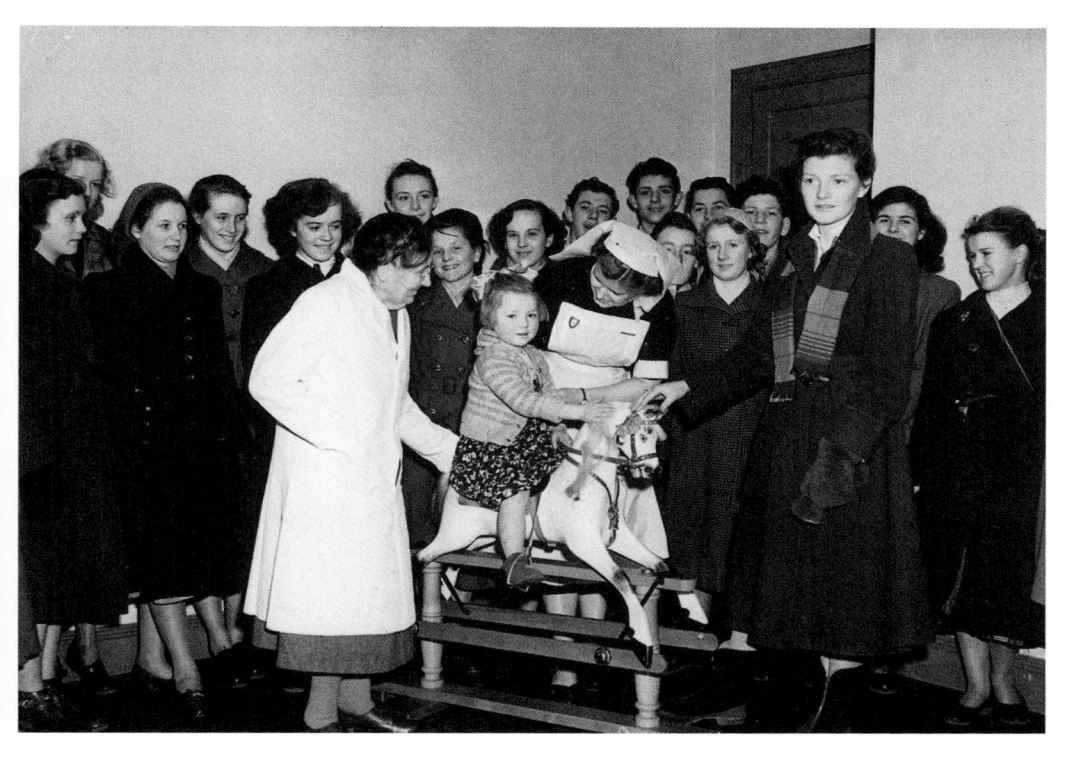

7. Child on a rocking horse with Dr. Lynn, a nurse and Rathmines Junior Red Cross, 1954. (Courtesy of the Royal College of Physicians of Ireland).

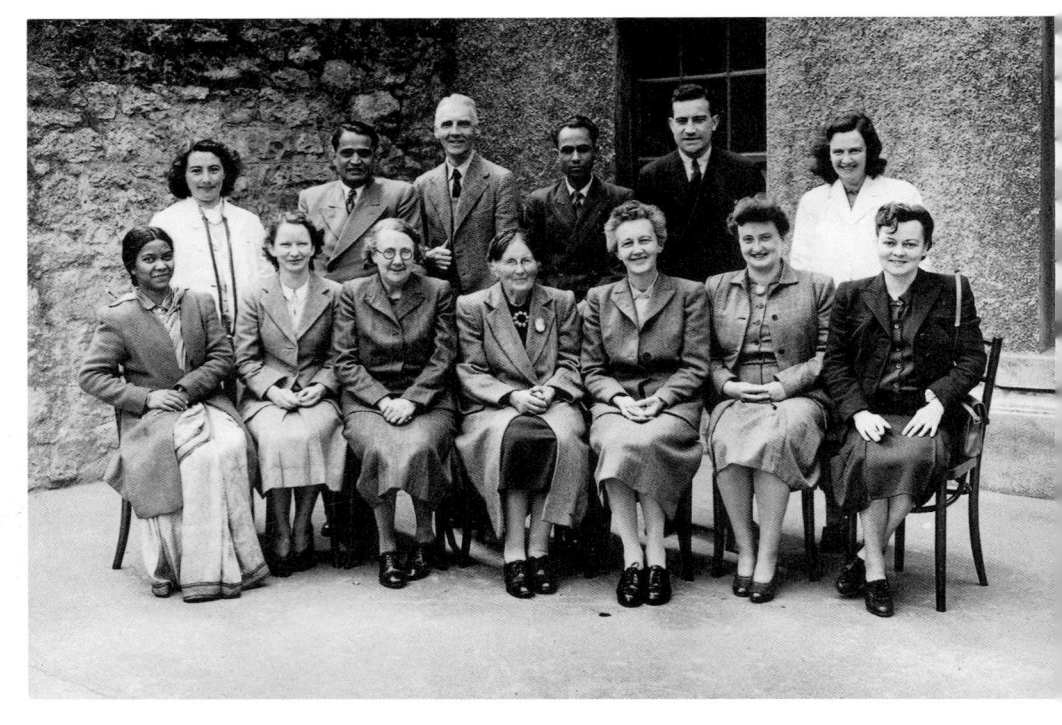

8. Postgraduate Course Participants and Staff of St. Ultan's, 1949. (Courtesy of the Royal College of Physicians of Ireland).

Cosgrave declared in 1923, during the Civil War, that 'women doctors and the clergy ought to keep out of politics, as their business is with the sick'.[103]

Lynn's political career faded as her involvement with St Ultan's took up most of her time. Was this an admission of failure or success in a different form? Perhaps Lynn, with her desire to influence, realised that she would have a greater impact in medicine than in politics. Like many others, she knew that socio-economic issues were ignored in the tense political environment of the 1920s. While there were conflicts over the Oath of Allegiance and advocates of pro- and anti-Treaty positions, 20,000 Dublin families lived in one-roomed tenements. In 1925, the City of Dublin Chief Medical Officer for Health, Dr M.J. Russell, suggested that bad housing was 'more responsible for the present high rate of infant mortality in Dublin than dirty milk'.[104] Lynn turned to these problems because she believed that children were future citizens of the new nation. In the 1920s, infant mortality ranged from 66 per 1,000 births, to 72 per 1,000. It would not dip below 50 until 1950.[105] The limitations of a small hospital were obvious. The Irish Free State continued to depend on voluntary groups (including religious orders) for welfare facilities. Ireland, both pre- and post-independence, was not noted for the emphasis it placed on social policy.[106] Political issues predominated. Meanwhile, in the words of Susanne Day, a member of the Cork Board of Guardians, 'slow murder by infection' was the fate of many.[107] Could Lynn and her colleagues stem this murderous tide?

In a work that examines American women in the professions, it was suggested that the early pioneers were 'apt to be women of extraordinary drive and commitment'. Their willingness to remain single and their superperformance were also highlighted.[108] Lynn is a classic example of this kind of activity. One month before St Ultan's opened, she wrote: 'Day busy as usual.'[109] Lynn would have many busy days at St Ultan's. As her political ambitions faded, she found professional fulfilment and frustration in St Ultan's, her medical republic.

Through medicine, Lynn expressed her own particular potent mix of patriotism and partisanship. However, in the 1930s, Lynn's medical republic was to face attacks from the ecclesiastical autocracy of the Roman Catholic Church and the medical profession. On the eve of the establishment of St Ultan's, the historian Alice Stopford Green suggested that 'round these tiny sufferers no question of politics or religion can arise'.[110] Nothing could be further from the truth. Lynn's aspirations would not be realised in the Irish Free State. Politics and sectarianism would triumph over compassion and justice.

NOTES

1 St Ultan's Annual Report, 1923.
2 Gisela Bock, 'Poverty and mothers' rights in the emerging welfare states' in Francoise Thébaud (ed.), *A History of Women in the West: volume V, Towards a Cultural Identity in the Twentieth Century* (Harvard, Cambridge and London, 1994), pp. 402–32, p. 403.
3 Jones, *The History of Tuberculosis in Nineteenth and Twentieth Century Ireland*, pp. 101–26, is an excellent start.
4 Joel Mokyr, 'Why "More Work for Mother?:" Knowledge and household behaviour, 1870–1945', in *The Journal of Economic History*, March 2000, vol. 60, no. 1, pp. 1–41, p. 9.
5 Lynn's second statement, Allen Library.
6 William Lawson, 'Infant mortality and the Notification of Births Acts, 1907, 1915', in *Journal of the Statistical and Social Inquiry Society of Ireland*, part xcvii, vol. xiii, Oct. 1919, pp. 479–97, p. 485.
7 Ida Blom, 'Equality and the threat of war in Scandinavia, 1884–1905', in T.G. Fraser and Keith Jeffery (eds), *Men, Women and War* (Dublin, 1993), pp. 100–18, p. 108.
8 *Alexandra College Magazine*, June 1908, p. 60.
9 Countess of Aberdeen, 'The Sphere of Women in Relation to Public Health' in *The Dublin Journal of Medical Science*, Sept. 1911, pp. 161–70.
10 *Golden Jubilee, 1907–1957: The Women's National Health Association of Ireland* (Dublin, 1957), pp. 1–12.
11 Lawson, 'Infant mortality' p. 487.
12 Janet Dunwoody, 'Child Welfare', in David Fitzpatrick (ed.), *Ireland and the First World War* (Dublin, 1986), pp. 69–75, p. 75.
13 Edward Coey Bigger, *The Carnegie United Kingdom Trust: Report on the Physical Welfare of Mothers and Children: vol. IV, Ireland, 1917* (Dublin, 1917), p. 9. Coey Bigger was the Medical Commissioner of the Local Government Board for Ireland.
14 Coey Bigger, *The Carnegie United Kingdom Trust*, p. 5. By contrast, the mortality rate per 1,000 for children under five in the Republic of Ireland in 2000 was 1.5 for males and 1.2 for females; Central Statistics Office, *Statistical Yearbook of Ireland, 2001* (Dublin, 2001), p. 45.

15 Charles A. Cameron, 'How the Dublin Poor Live', in *Reminiscences of Sir Charles A. Cameron, C.B.* (Dublin and London, 1913), pp. 165–67, p. 165.
16 Between 1913 and 1923 infant mortality was 99 per 1,000 in urban areas and 50 in rural areas; William Thompson, 'A Few Outstanding Points in Connection with the Vital Statistics of the Irish Free State' in *Irish Journal of Medical Science*, April 1925, pp. 145–61, p. 150.
17 Marjorie Perrin Behringer, 'Women's role and status in the sciences: an historical perspective', in Jane Butler Kahle (ed.), *Women in Science: A Report from the Field* (Philadelphia, 1985), pp. 4–26, p. 17.
18 First Minute Book of St Ultan's, 18 July 1918, SUA.
19 1926 Irish Free State Census.
20 Ministry of Health, Annual Report of the Chief Medical Officer, 1919–1920 vol. xvii, 1920, Cmd.978, p. 155; *Annual Reports of the Board of Superintendence of the Dublin Hospitals, with Appendices*, 1920–21 p. 5; 1921–22, p. 5; 1922–23, p. 8.
21 The information on St Ultan is taken from the Annual Reports of the Hospital. He was a kinsman of St Brigid, whom Lynn admired. Ultan wrote a hymn to St Brigid, see Angela Bourke, Siobhán Kilfeather, Maria Luddy, Margaret MacCurtain, Gerardine Meaney, Máirín Ní Dhonnchadha, Mary O'Dowd and Clair Wills (eds), *The Field Day Anthology of Irish Writing: vol. IV: Irish Women's Writing and Traditions* (Cork, 2002), pp. 62–3.
22 LD, 15 August 1919; Ó hÓgartaigh, Margaret, 'St Ultan and Ardbraccan' in *Ríocht na Midhe: Records of the Meath Archaeological and Historical Society*, vol. xiv, 2003, pp. 230–41. Lynn also enjoyed visiting Mother Columba Gibbons in Co. Meath, see Margaret Ó hÓgartaigh, 'Mother Columba Gibbons of the Loreto Convent in Navan and author of the ballad "Who fears to speak of Easter Week"', in *Ríocht na Midhe: Records of the Meath Archaeological and Historical Society*, vol. xvi, 2005, pp. 189–93.
23 *Alexandra College Magazine*, June 1898, pp. 258–61; Maryann Gialanella Valiulis, 'Toward "The Moral and Material Improvement of the Working Classes: The Founding of the Alexandra College Guild Tenement Company, Dublin, 1898, *Journal of Urban History*, vol. 23, no. 3, March 1997, pp. 295–314; Mitchell, *Adelaide*, p. 111; *Alexandra College Magazine*, Jan. 1893, p. 38; *British Medical Journal*, 22 August 1931.
24 Belfast Eugenics Society Minutes in Queen's University Belfast, Special Collections, MS 66/1; Greta Jones, 'Eugenics in Ireland: The Belfast Eugenics Society', in *Irish Historical Studies*, vol. xxviii, no. 109, (May 1992), pp. 81–95.
25 I am grateful to the Dictionary of Irish Biography and Frances Clarke, in particular, for details on Alice Barry. She also features prominently in the SUA. For Barry's divisive activities at St Ultan's, see chapter 4.
26 Kirkpatrick Biographical Archive; *Irish Independent*, 10 Feb. 1938; *Irish Times*, 10 Feb. 1938.
27 A brief summary of Dr Webb's career is available in Mitchell *Adelaide*, pp. 260–62. However, it contains several errors. For example, he notes that she

was awarded her MD in 1925 (the RUI Calendar indicates it was 1906) and he also suggests that she only became involved in St Ultan's after her husband's death in 1929. The St Ultan's minutes have several references to the Webbs working in the hospital in the early 1920s. Kirkpatrick Biographical Archive; *Irish Times*, 26 Aug. 1946; *Irish Times*, 27 Aug. 1946; *Irish Press*, 26 Aug. 1946; *Lancet*, 4 June 1916; *British Medical Journal*, 7 Sept. 1946.

28 *St Stephen's*, Nov. 1904, p. 111.
29 *Alexandra College Magazine*, June 1924, p. 33.
30 *Irish Times*, 27 Aug. 1946.
31 Typescript entitled 'Teach [Ultáin] History Notes', SUA.
32 LD, 9 March 1921.
33 Unfortunately, and revealingly, the St Ultan's Annual Reports do not give us the names of the nurses. Despite being an all-female institution, the traditional hierarchies of Irish hospitals, with the contribution of nurses muted, persisted in St Ultan's. On nursing, see Margaret Ó hÓgartaigh, 'Flower Power and "Mental Grooviness": nurses and midwives in Ireland in the early twentieth century', in Whelan (ed.), *Women and Paid Work in Ireland, 1500–1930*, pp. 133–47.
34 First Minute Book of St Ultan's, 19 Mar. 1918 SUA
35 First Minute Book of St Ultan's, 2 May and 9 Apr. 1918, SUA.
36 First Minute Book of St Ultan's, 7 Nov., 30 Nov. and 30 Dec. 1918, SUA; LD, 29 May 1919.
37 St Ultan's Annual Report 1926; St Ultan's Annual Report 1922, p. 8
38 LD, 3 Oct. 1919.
39 Second Minute Book, but First Official Minute Book of St Ultan's (hereafter Official Minute Book), 15 Sept. 1921; newspaper cuttings, September 1923, in ffrench-Mullen scrapbooks, courtesy of the Murphy family.
40 Typescript entitled *Teach [Ultáin] History Notes*, SUA.
41 St Ultan's Official Minute Book, 20 Jan. and 20 Oct., 1921, SUA.
42 St Ultan's Official Minute Book, 17 Nov., 1921, SUA.
43 Newspapers cuttings, no specific sources cited, Nov–April 1920–21, ffrench-Mullen scrapbook. Eileen ffrench-Mullen later became a Carmelite nun.
44 26 May 1927, in ffrench-Mullen scrapbook, no newspaper cited. *Irish Times*, 16 Dec. 1928; *Irish Independent*, 17 August 1928. The Irish White Cross gave £1,623 according to the St Ultan's Annual Report 1921, p. 8.
45 *Irish Nursing News*, Oct. 1928, insert in ffrench-Mullen scrapbook; I.A. Abt was the author of 'Influenza in a newly born infant', in *Journal of the American Medical Association*, 1919, no. 72, pp. 980–81, and he edited *Abt-Garrison history of paediatrics* (Philadelphia, 1965). For a comprehensive history of infant care, see Murdina MacFarquhar Desmond, *Newborn Medicine and Society: European Background and American Practice (1750–1975)* (Austin, 1998). I am grateful to the author for giving me a copy of her book.
46 Dr Kathleen Lynn, 'The milk and the murder of babies', in *Old Ireland*, 21 August 1920, pp. 449–50.

47 'Breastfeeding and infant mortality', in *British Medical Journal*, August 2001, abstract in *The International Journal of Clinical Medicine, Modern Medicine of Ireland*, vol. 31, no. 10, October 2001, p. 66.
48 Typescript entitled *Teach [Ultáin] History Notes* in SUA.
49 *The Irish Times*, [no precise date given] December 1924, ffrench-Mullen scrapbook.
50 Coey Bigger, *The Carnegie United Kingdom Trust*. pp. 45–6.
51 Typescript entitled 'Teach [Ultáin] History Notes' in SUA; St Ultan's Annual Report 1923.
52 Cited in Jane Lewis, *The Politics of Motherhood: Child and Maternal Welfare in England, 1900–1939* (London, 1980), pp. 89 and 92.
53 Isabel Magill, 'A social history of T.B. in Belfast' (D.Phil., University of Ulster at Jordanstown, 1992), p. 67.
54 William Thompson, 'A few outstanding points in connection with the vital statistics of the Irish Free State', in *Irish Journal of Medical Science*, April 1925, pp. 145–61, p. 151. Terminology specific to the period in question is used in order to avoid ahistorical terms, hence the use of the word 'illegitimate'.
55 Article on St Ultan's by Edla Wortabet in *The British Journal of Nursing* 23 Oct. 1920, ffrench-Mullen scrapbook.
56 Insert on St Ultan's week, the first anniversary of the hospital, ffrench-Mullen Scrapbook.
57 *Irish Independent*, 2 June 1919, ffrench-Mullen Scrapbook.
58 Newspaper insert in ffrench-Mullen scrapbook, 1922. No specific source cited.
59 Letter is dated 6 May 1922, and the handwritten heading is 'The Irish Republic of Chicago', ffrench-Mullen scrapbook.
60 Lynn to ffrench-Mullen, 7 and 9 Dec. 1922, Captured Documents Lot 120, Military Archives, Cathal Brugha Barracks, Dublin.
61 No newspaper cited, 1924 ffrench-Mullen Scrapbook.
62 *Honesty*, 13 June 1925, ffrench-Mullen Scrapbook.
63 National Children's Hospital [Harcourt Street] Annual Report 1928, p. 16.
64 19 April 1923, no newspaper cited, ffrench-Mullen Scrapbook.
65 Reports of Registrar General, 1926–30.
66 Medical Committee, 15 October 1922, SUA. The Medical Committee of St Ultan's usually met once a month. Drs Magure, Lynn, Tennant and Barry, with Webb in the chair, constituted the medical committee.
67 Medical Committee, 17 January 1923, SUA.
68 Medical Committee, 10 February 1926, SUA.
69 St Ultan's Annual Report 1926 p. 8; LD 7 March 1919; St Ultan's Annual Reports 1925–1935.
70 Ruth McManus, *Dublin, 1910–1940: Shaping the City & Suburbs* (Dublin, 2002), pp. 269–73.
71 Discussions regarding the flats were regular items on the agenda in the 1940s, see St Ultan's General Committee Minutes, SUA. See also chapter 5 for details.
72 Dr Liam Ó Sé, discussion at the Royal Academy of Medicine in Ireland, 16 October 2002.

73 *Irish Nursing News*, Dec. 1928, p. 37.
74 Cited in Lewis, *The Politics of Motherhood*, p. 92.
75 LD, 6 March 1924.
76 The group included Dr Charles Mayo of the Mayo Clinic, *Irish Times*, 11 June 1925, ffrench-Mullen Scrapbook.
77 LD, 7 August 1925.
78 Lynn to Matthew Russell, 3 November 1925, in Rockefeller Archives, Sleepy Hollow, New York State. My thanks to Melissa Kafes for making my trip to the Rockefeller Archives so fruitful.
79 For details on Lynn's activities in New York see LD October and November 1925, and USA Medical Directories for the 1920s, Emerson's book is in the Countway Medical Library, Harvard University.
80 No newspaper cited, Jan–May 1926, ffrench-Mullen Scrapbook.
81 Ellen S. More, *Restoring the Balance: Women Physicians and the Profession of Medicine, 1850–1995* (Cambridge, Mass. and London, 1999), p. 74; LD, 6 Nov. 1925; Margaret Ó hÓgartaigh, 'The Babies' Clubs in Ireland and the Children's Bureau in the US', in Chester Burns, Ynez Violé O'Neill, Philippe Albou and José Gabriel Rigau-Pérez (eds) *Proceedings of the 37th International Congress on the History of Medicine* (Galveston, Texas, 2001), pp. 99–103.
82 *Irish Independent*, 28 May 1926.
83 St Ultan's Annual Report 1927, p. 16.
84 St Ultan's Annual Report 1930, p. 6.
85 LD, 21 March 1920.
86 LD, 2, 5 and 20 Oct. 1920.
87 LD, 24 April 1921.
88 LD, 17 March 1925.
89 LD, 24 and 26 Dec. 1920.
90 LD, 27 Dec. 1920.
91 Fanny Ceannt to Lily O'Brennan [her sister], 10 April 1923, UCDA O'Brennan Papers, P13/52.
92 LD, 7 and 8 April 1923.
93 LD, 18 Feb. 1919.
94 LD 25 Sept. 1919.
95 Interview with Dr Dónal Caird, who knew Lynn through Cumann Gaelach na hEaglaise in the 1940s, June 2000.
96 LD, 3 Nov. 1923.
97 LD, 10 March 1924.
98 LD, 19 May 1926.
99 According to William Wynne, a relation of the Lynn family, Muriel was a committed Unionist and refused to live in the Irish Free State.
100 LD, 29 Dec. 1926.
101 LD, 19 Dec. 1924.
102 Cited in Anderson, *Connolly and the Irish Left*, p. 76.
103 Cited in Anderson, *Connolly and the Irish Left*, p. 81.
104 *Irish Times*, 29 May 1925; the article, entitled 'Child Mortality', was an examination of St Ultan's work.

105 Figures from the Annual Reports of the Registrar General.
106 Maria Maguire, 'The Development of the Welfare State in Ireland in the Postwar Period' (Ph.D., European University Institute, 1985), p. 2.
107 Susanne Day, *The Amazing Philanthropists* (London, 1916), p. 35; Bourke et al., *Field Day Anthology of Irish Writing*, pp. 88–91. Day, like Lynn, was interested in suffrage as well as reforming the treatment of the vulnerable.
108 Penina Migdal Glazer and Miriam Slater, *Unequal Colleagues: The Entrance of Women into the Professions, 1890–1940* (London, 1987), pp. 69 and 85.
109 LD, 10 April 1919.
110 *Evening Herald*, 17 May 1919.

CHAPTER FOUR

The politics of children's health, 1928–39

IN 1956 AN ÓIGE (the Youth) Hostel in Glenmalure, County Wicklow and Our Lady's Hospital for Sick Children in Crumlin, Dublin were opened. Both events were connected to Lynn and their origins lay in the 1930s. The Irish Free State of the 1930s is associated with faith and fatherland. The 1930s also saw the reinforcement of women's traditional roles. This idealisation of female virtue and modesty placed faith and motherhood at the core of an increasingly Catholic-centred nation. What did this mean for radical women like Lynn? Their work both in the public and private arenas was carefully scrutinised. The very fact that Lynn's work focused on women and children brought her into conflict with the Catholic Church which closely monitored the activities of philanthropic organisations.

Much work has been done on Catholic social thinking and its implications in the newly emerging state.[1] This had particular implications for women and children. Diocesan archivist, David Sheehy, perceptively pointed out that the 'profession of the Catholic Church is women and children'.[2] Thus, great emphasis was placed on the alleged sanctity of the family. After independence, 'children were not afforded the same status that they had been given in the Democratic Programme of the first Dáil in 1919 which had placed the care of children as "the first duty of the republic" whereas the Constitution of 1937 sought to protect "the family" from interference by the state'.[3] Hence, families were seen as sacrosanct. These ideals meant that someone involved in child care and the improvement of children's health, as Lynn was, would clash with ecclesiastical and secular authorities.

This chapter will examine the consolidation of Lynn's professional career as well as her republican activities. Her progressive approach to the care of infants in evident is the links between Dr Maria Montessori and St Ultan's. The proposed amalgamation of the National Children's Hospital on Harcourt Street and St Ultan's brought Lynn and her colleagues into conflict with Drs Byrne and McQuaid, the Roman Catholic Archbishops. It can be argued that Lynn's approach directly contradicted the ideological imperatives of the new state. Her response to national developments, such as the 1937 Constitution, and international events, such as the rise of Fascism, were conditioned by her commitment to feminism and socialism. Hence, both nationally and internationally, she was a critic of the state. Furthermore, as a member of a religious minority she was seen as suspect in the eyes of certain Catholics. Her approach to medicine posed a threat both real and imagined to the organisation of medical provision in Ireland.

There were particular concerns about upholding Catholic values in the new state. The *Catholic Bulletin* asked: 'Is the School of Medicine, Trinity College, Dublin, a safe place for the training of doctors who are to practise, even to practise with the prestige [of] a civil appointment, among the Catholic people of Ireland, poor or rich?'[4] Protestants were seen as posing a moral threat to Catholics. Lynn was to be affected by these views, particularly after the 1930 Church of England Lambeth Conference, which approved of birth control in certain circumstances.[5] Much has been written about Letitia Dunbar-Harrison, like Lynn, a female Protestant, whose appointment as librarian in Mayo caused a furore as it was suggested that a Protestant could not be trusted with Catholic clients.[6] However, the subtext to this incident was the presence of a local candidate, Miss Burke, who had failed to be appointed. Occasionally, Catholic ethics were a disguise which hid the desire to appoint the local candidate. There was at least one medical Dunbar-Harrison case. In the mid 1920s, sectarian arguments were used in Kilskyne, County Meath when a Catholic female, Dr Eileen Brangan, was passed over for a local appointment in favour of Dr Francis O'Brien-Kennedy, a Protestant outsider. The Vicar General 'drew attention to the fact that religion formed an important element in the appointment of a dispensary doctor'.[7] However, the appointment was not changed. Jack White has suggested that a system of 'apartheid' existed in Irish hospitals, with private hospitals 'controlled by voluntary and largely self-perpetuating boards of governors'.[8]

These incidents revealed the fear of Protestant practices and resentment over their perceived, and sometimes real, socio-economic advantages. Dr Gilmartin, the Catholic Bishop of Tuam, quoted statute 256 of canon law, which enjoined the parish priest to ensure that 'the Faithful, especially midwives, doctors and surgeons, learn well the correct manner of conferring Baptism in the case of necessity'. The following statute (257) was even more emphatic and would have profound implications for Protestant doctors:

> Parish Priests and other priests are bound to prevent the impious crime by which, through the aid of surgical instruments or other means, the infant is killed in the womb. Wherefore let them use their best efforts to have deputed to public positions only those doctors and surgeons who have prosecuted their studies in schools where Catholic principles in this matter are recognised.[9]

Economics triumphed over ideology. However, Catholic ethics aroused considerable debate. All of these concerns have to be borne in mind when considering the difficulties faced by Lynn in the 1930s.

PROPOSED NEW CHILDREN'S HOSPITAL

The medical care of infants was not given a high priority by the medical profession in general. Several authors noted that paediatrics did not occupy a high place in the medical hierarchy. Dr Robert (Bob) Collis, writing of the 1930s, suggested that the 'position of paediatrics at that moment in Dublin was very much at its beginnings and the prospects of being able to support oneself rather slim'.[10] One Trinity academic described paediatrics as a 'notifiable disease'.[11] However, Dr Pearl Dunlevy, who was heavily involved in the BCG vaccination campaign (which helped eliminate tuberculosis) in the 1950s, believed that jobs were easier to obtain in paediatrics.[12]

Throughout the 1920s and '30s, Lynn bemoaned the presence of so many sick infants. In 1932, infant mortality in Ireland was 72 per

1,000. In Dublin, it was a shocking 100 per 1,000.[13] In other words, of every 100 infants born in Dublin, ten would not see their first birthday. There was a great need for a large children's hospital in Dublin. The medical committee of St Ultan's reported in 1934 that the death rate at the hospital had dropped from 33.5 per cent to 22 per cent.[14] Clearly, while progress was being made improved facilities were needed. Within a couple of months the plans for a new hospital were 'considered in detail'. Michael Scott, the well-known architect and Lynn's friend, had presented plans for the hospital which would be built along by the canal.[15] St Ultan's would amalgamate with Harcourt Children's Hospital in order to provide a proper paediatric service. This was Lynn's dream. What was most frustrating about her work was seeing older children come to St Ultan's outpatient department obviously in need of medical aid but with nowhere to go. Along with Dr Elizabeth Tennant, Lynn represented St Ultan's on the Joint Committee for the amalgamation of Harcourt Street and St Ultan's.[16]

Lynn was a dominant figure on both the general board and the medical committee of St Ultan's and she was determined to have her own way. Her persistence led to financial negotiations with solicitors, accountants and welfare officers, not to mention local government officials. However, the slow pace of developments frequently frustrated her. Lack of money, for once, was not the problem. The Hospitals' Sweepstakes was very generous in its funding for St Ultan's.[17] In 1930 they received £14,000 from this source.[18] Indeed, Sir Joseph Glynn, Vice-Chairman of the Hospitals' Sweeps Committee, declared at the 1935 Annual General Meeting of the hospital that 'women were the backbone of any movement for the health of the people'.[19] It was the Hospitals' Commission which suggested that St Ultan's and Harcourt Street become a joint hospital. St Ultan's agreed in principle but they declared that the 'objects of this special hospital would have to be safeguarded'.[20] The independent-minded women who had established St Ultan's did not want to lose control of their hospital. Lynn was to realise that optimistic plans could be scuppered by political considerations.

During the 1930s, the diaries of Lynn are filled with aspirations for the future. Because money was suddenly available for hospital expansion through the Hospitals' Sweepstakes, it raised hopes for an improvement in the medical provisions for infants. However, the Sweepstakes could be a Trojan horse for increased state involvement in medicine. 'Over the succeeding decades the lines of cooperation with, and dependence on the state, became increasingly blurred and consequently all the more ferociously guarded.'[21]

AMALGAMATION OF THE NATIONAL CHILDREN'S HOSPITAL AT HARCOURT STREET AND ST ULTAN'S

St Ultan's, as noted earlier, was the only hospital in Ireland managed, though not staffed, entirely by women. Furthermore, these women were multi-denominational. One could argue that the experiences of St Ultan's in general, and Lynn, in particular, reflected broader trends in society, specifically, the denominational organisation of Irish medicine. Lynn was to become entangled in these tensions and her helplessness and frustration are all the more poignant given the implications of the delay for patients.

For Lynn, 1930 had begun well with the donation of $1,051 from Anna Smith as part of the Christmas appeal in New York.[22] In the 1930s St Ultan's was to have strained relations with Dr Edward Byrne, the Roman Catholic Archbishop of Dublin. One of the constant difficulties facing St Ultan's was the lack of space. There was a grave shortage of paediatric beds. Furthermore, hospitals were either under Protestant or Catholic management. St Ultan's was perceived as a Protestant hospital since it was not under Catholic control. Partly for socio-economic reasons, and partly due to patronage, Protestants were over-represented in the medical profession. This created professional tensions and jealousies. Attempts in the 1920s by the Rockefeller Foundation to generously fund the development of clinical education were scuppered by petty jealousies and rivalries, in particular between TCD and UCD.[23] Revealingly, Trinity saw itself as the bastion of accumulated medical knowledge, since its School of Physic dated from the eighteenth century. Moreover, the mono-denominational organisation of medicine and education was exacerbated by the desire of the new state to make reparations for discrimination and injustices suffered under British rule. Mary E. Daly has noted that 'sectarian divisions' were evident in the development of hospital care. Sean T. O'Kelly, Minister for Local Government and Public Health, suggesting that Protestants were favoured over Catholics in appointments, 'noted that "NUI men" [graduates of the National University] did not get a fair share of appointments in the hospitals which were in receipt of government grants: most of the medical staff were graduates of Trinity College, Dublin'.[24] Furthermore, when the Hospitals' Sweepstakes were being discussed in the Dáil in 1930, Fianna Fáil wanted to omit hospitals which it believed discriminated on religious grounds.[25]

These arguments would also be aired when St Ultan's was attempting to amalgamate with Harcourt Street. Like St Ultan's, Harcourt Street was not under Catholic management, hence it aroused the suspicion of ecclesiastics like Dr Byrne and Dr John Charles McQuaid, then President of Blackrock College, a prominent boys' secondary school managed by the Holy Ghost Fathers.

The proposed amalgamation between St Ultan's and Harcourt Street aroused accusations of sterilisation and sex education. The controversy was orchestrated by McQuaid, articulated by Byrne, and fortified by the energetic efforts of Catholic correspondents such as Drs Stafford Johnson and Marie Lea-Wilson. Both of these medical practitioners conducted sectarian audits of Dublin hospitals and noted the number of Catholic and Protestant physicians working in various institutions. Stafford Johnson was a leading light in the Knights of Columbanus, a Masonic-like organisation which promoted Catholic values and sought opportunities for Catholic professionals.[26] Interestingly, Stafford Johnson was a great friend of McQuaid and always accompanied him on his holidays to Rockwell College, a Holy Ghost school in south Tipperary.[27] He was also one of the founder members of the Irish Guild of SS Luke, Cosmos and Damian. One of its aims was to 'promote amongst Catholic members of the profession such solidarity as may be of advantage both to their religion and their profession'.[28] Professional ambitions chimed most conveniently with ethical aspirations. Lea-Wilson had trained as a doctor after the murder of her husband at the hands of the IRA. She worked in

Harcourt Street, the National Children's Hospital, which was not under Catholic management.[29] Finola Kennedy, whose mother, Dr Nora Stack, was a friend of Lea-Wilson, thought she was a 'devout and pious Catholic' who was dedicated to the welfare of Polish and Russian Catholics.[30]

While the medical profession indulged in professional politics, infants died. Lynn's diaries are a poignant reminder of the futility of her plans. At the beginning of 1935 she was hopeful: 'Dr Barry says amalgamation with Harcourt Street would be very good'. Yet, the following day she wrote, 'Dr Trevor Smith [who worked in the Royal Hospital for Incurables, Donnybrook] came to tell me privately what a dreadful person Dr Collis was.'[31] Bob Collis worked in Harcourt Street and was very interested in social medicine. He was to expose the dreadful social conditions of the Dublin tenements through his controversial play *Marrowbone Lane*. When Collis founded the Irish Paediatric Club in 1933 (it later became the Irish Paediatric Association), its first meeting was held at Dr Price's home in 10 Fitzwilliam Place. Lynn and Ella Webb also attended the inaugural meeting.[32] Collis was a colleague of Dr Marie Lea-Wilson, and made no secret of his dislike for her. In his autobiography he described her as follows: 'she was the strongest character I have ever met, a lady of indomitable force who literally could not be stopped if she decided on a course of action. She had worked herself into an invaluable position in the hospital [Harcourt Street] by years as a house officer . . . she had no special degrees, and was not a real paediatrician at all. But she personally interviewed every member of the Board with such vigour that when it came to the actual election the Board was unable to choose between us.'[33] The board chose all three candidates. This may be professional pique on the part of Collis. However, there were individuals in both institutions who were wary of amalgamation.

Meanwhile, Lynn was in contact with the architect Michael Scott who was 'delighted with amalgamation proposal'.[34] All was not serene at St Ultan's though, and Lynn admitted that while the general board did not 'disapprove of Principle of Amalgamation', the members were not enthusiastic. More prophetically, she asked, 'Dr [Alice] Barry is always thorny now, why?'[35] A week later she bemoaned the fact that St Ultan's was 'full of bad babies'.[36] It was a common complaint. That summer Lynn wrote that 'the amount of sick babies is appalling, I never remembered more. Teac goes well in spite of all.'[37] By the autumn, she was beginning to realise that there was a lot of opposition to the amalgamation but she remained hopeful.

What gave rise to opposition to the amalgamation? Ecclesiastical politics obviously played a part. In November, it was revealed that Edward Byrne had become embroiled in the issue. Lynn wrote, 'Medical Board went well. Dr Barry only objected to amalgamation because we hadn't beds enough! No word of Dr Byrne (Archbishop) Dr P[rice] says Moorhead only approached by Stafford Johnston on subject, never by Archbishop. It is all mean, underhand work.'[38] The issue had become contentious.

It is clear from the minutes of the St Ultan's Medical Board and the General Committee that there were deep divisions at the hospital. A sectarian divide was developing. The medical board was dominated by Drs Price, Lynn, Webb, Tennant (all of whom were Protestant), and Barry seems to have been the only person on the board who wished to comply with the views of the Archbishop. On the other hand, the General Committee was more mixed, with 50/50 Catholic/Protestant representation. At a special meeting of the St Ultan's General Committee in November, there were references to Dr Byrne, and 'Dr Barry stated that she did not approve of the proposed constitution' which would formalise the link between Harcourt Street and St Ultan's. Dr Tennant suggested that the meeting 'await the report of the medical board'. This amendment was put to the meeting and lost. Significantly, Lynn wanted to know what way people were voting. Her distress and frustration are evident, yet she remained hopeful: 'Dr Barry proposed turning down report of Co-ordination Committee and it was carried, 8 votes to 5. She saw her party had majority and forced vote. But we, who have worked always for Teac, are not disheartened. God will show the way out we know.'[39] At a special meeting of the medical board in November 1935, matters came to a head. Barry was not representing the views of the medical board on the General Committee. It was therefore proposed by Price and seconded by Lynn, that she resign as a representative of the medical board.[40] That evening Lynn wrote: 'it went better than we thought thank God and we were all sorry we had to ask Dr Barry to resign off Medical Board when she should not consciously represent us for she holds that her Archbishop doesn't approve of amalgamation so she can't.'[41] Lynn's disgust at what had happened was apparent. 'We got out whole petty story of the Catholic Archbishop's disapproval, no reason given but that of religion which doesn't come in at all.'[42] As ever religion was the guise under which control could be exerted. The whole saga exhausted Lynn. At the end of November, she noted wearily: 'Such a day! Board meeting very full. I think both sides thought mobilised by the other, but no. It was a draw and now there is to be still another meeting on Monday 9th, it was very trying, bandying same old arguments. Dr Barry's party quite unmoved.'[43]

BRYNE'S CONCERNS

Eventually, in December 1935, at a special meeting of the General Committee, it was decided to send a deputation to Dr Byrne, the Roman Catholic Archbishop. Lynn suggested that it was 'as well to get definite reasons from him regarding his alleged opposition'.[44] Afterwards, she complained: 'Archbishop gave long list of his "reasons" against amalgamation, all the things we have never done and can easily say will never be done, he is terrible, domineering without reason. We can well answer all he says. We know right will prevail D.G.'[45] Dr Byrne wrote to St Ultan's Hospital in December, 1935. His opposition was very revealing: 'I oppose this amalgamation on religious principles solely. I consider that in such a united institution the Faith of Catholic children (who will be 99% of the total treated) would not be safe. The Faith of Catholic children is of more importance in the eyes of the Catholic Church than any other thing in the world.' In order to emphasise his point Dr Byrne quoted Cardinal Newman. 'The Church would rather save the soul of one person than carry out a sanitary reform, in its fullest details, in every city in Sicily.' Was this ecclesiastical bluster or a genuine focus on the missionary role of Catholics? Whatever the reason, the grim reality of infant ill health was seen as less important than denominational control.

Byrne reiterated his opposition to the merger for the following reasons: the amalgamation

> 'would create a virtual monopoly in the medical treatment of children in the south side of the city. This monopoly is to be ceded to a body whose whole attitude to the Catholic view-point would be at least suspect and I fear even hostile. During the past few months both hospitals have proved that there is a body of opinion in them unwilling to meet Catholic objections to amalgamation. Examples of this may be found in the statement attributed to Dr Moorhead . . . that the Archbishop of Dublin has "no status" and in the resignation of Dr Barry, called for and effected on November 20th. Clearly, the atmosphere of the amalgamated institution would be over-whelmingly non-Catholic and in such an institution Catholic children, who would form 99% of the patients, would find themselves in a predominantly non-Catholic atmosphere. To this I will never consent.'

Because children up to 16 years would be catered for, Byrne asked: 'how can we view without alarm the proposed establishment of a centre of Paediatrics in an institution predominantly unsympathetic to Catholic teaching.' Ethics were also an issue. 'A children's hospital catering for children from infancy to 16 years is concerned with the many serious and delicate problems of puberty and pre-adolescent stage. The danger of naturalistic and wrong teachings on sex instruction or adolescent problems is a powerful argument for retaining the custody of children in Catholic hands.' These issues should not be seen in isolation: there was an active Marie Stopes Clinic which offered contraceptive advice in Belfast during the 1930s. Furthermore, Professor T.G. Moorhead, in a talk to the Dublin University Law Society at Trinity College on 'Insanity and Criminal Law', proposed that the 'criminally-minded insane' and 'habitual offenders should be sterilised'. Moreover, he argued that the 'progeny of mental defectives are more likely to be affected (by a tendency towards crime)'.[46] These ideas were far from new in the 1930s, but they were anathema for devout Catholics.

Byrne had obviously read the report of Moorhead's talk: 'There is a widespread attack on Catholic morals through the medium of medicine.' He suggested that 'Trinity College [would] be the dominating influence in the Paediatric centre of the amalgamated hospitals.' Even more damning, 'contraceptive practices are recommended by many non-Catholic doctors. The outpatient dept of a children's hospital provided a possible place for advocating such practices.' Souperism also raised its ugly head. 'There is increased social activity by many non-Catholics directed towards the care of children in many directions. It is a matter of common knowledge that proselytism is rife and that Catholics have been obliged to spend money and take active measures to safeguard the Catholic Faith of unfortunate mothers and their children.' There were fears in Ireland that poor children would be encouraged to change their faith. The Smyly Homes, which catered for Protestant orphans, were accused of proselytism. Finally, Byrne prophesised: 'what Harcourt Street now is we may expect the united hospitals will be when the solid non-Catholic Committee of Harcourt St is joined the to non-Catholic minority' of St Ultan's.[47]

Clearly the ghost of Mrs Smyly lingered. Furthermore, fascist regimes, particularly in Germany, *were* sterilising so-called 'mental defectives'. The concerns of Byrne have to be seen in this context.

ST ULTAN'S RESPONSE

Almost immediately St Ultan's replied to these allegations, in January 1936. They suggested that there was 'an entire misconception' as to the proposed hospital. 'There is no proposal before us to provide educational facilities, the hospital is to be for acute not chronic cases,' they replied. 'Sterilisation of the unfit does not come under the heading of children under 16 years'. In addition, they emphasised that they had 'never advocated birth control and have no intention of doing so in the future'. The Board of the National Children's Hospital is not 'solidly non-Catholic', since there is a Catholic matron and the majority of the nurses are Catholic. (However, most of the physicians were Protestant.) They assured Byrne that the 'Faith of the Children will not be tampered with'. Finally, they suggested that Dr Moorhead was 'not a paediatrician'.[48] This was true but he was a mentor for both Price and Lynn. Moorhead was seen as suspect by the 'Catholic actionists'. At the same time Lynn took matters into her own hands and wrote to Byrne as a 'private individual'.[49] She pointed out that in the 'proposed amalgamated hospital there is no idea of either religious or secular instruction being given', as the children would only be in the hospital for a short period. Moreover, she made it quite clear that none of the St Ultan's medical staff 'have ever heard of, much less practised, the giving of instruction in sex matters or birth control'. Lynn also pointed out that

> there is strong and growing objection to birth control among medical men and women. Dame Louise McIlroy, a Presbyterian from the north of Ireland, & Professor of obstetrics in London wrote very strongly condemning such practices a short while ago in the British Medical Journal. I myself, and many others not belonging to your flock, consider such practices immoral.

Lynn's comments are revealing of her attitude but it was very impolitic to mention Dr McIlroy. Her clinic at the Royal Free Hospital in London offered birth control advice.[50] This was exactly the kind of ammunition that Byrne and McQuaid used against Lynn and her colleagues. Furthermore, McIlroy had visited St Ultan's on a number of occasions. Determined forces were at work in order to prevent the establishment of a multi-denominational children's hospital. In 1936, the energetic and able Dr John Charles McQuaid, then president of Blackrock College, pronounced his dissatisfaction with the proposed amalgamation. McQuaid was to become a dynamic and controversial Archbishop of Dublin in 1940. Like Lynn he was very determined, highly intelligent and deeply aware of the great poverty in Dublin.[51] However, unlike Lynn he was resolutely unecumenical and depressingly suspicious of individuals he liked to describe as 'non-catholic'. McQuaid's letter to Byrne was inscribed 'by hand Secret'. He declared that Moorhead 'was doing his utmost to bring about amalgamation of Harcourt St and St Ultan's to prevent the Archbishop building his new Children's Hospital, that failing amalgamation he was working hard for the very large extension of St Ultan's with same purpose of blocking his Grace's scheme'. In order to make his point even clearer McQuaid warned Byrne, 'Moorhead is and remains the (venomous) spear-head of the Masonic opposition. I knew he was not idle, but he took a long time to declare his plans.' In conclusion, McQuaid warned that no time should be lost in countering the actions of Moorhead.[52]

The episode soured Lynn's relationship with institutional Catholicism, even though she had many Catholic friends. 'Our Abp. gets Gt. praise for counselling us all to take our part in the common life of the country & not be a garrison any longer. Press & Govt. v. pleased. A v. different tune fr. the R.C. Abp. who wouldn't let us live at all.'[53] As a member of a minority religion, Lynn did not fit the image of the independent Irish state. The ultimate losers, of course, were the children who needed medical help, and Lynn knew this. At a medical committee meeting in April 1936 'comments were made on the loss of life amongst cases which had to be refused admission for lack of accommodation'.[54]

Staffing was also an issue when the large Catholic children's hospital was built in Crumlin. In the Byrne papers there is a memorandum on the New Children's Hospital by Dr Stafford Johnson. He suggested that graduates of the National University should be employed in the hospital. The NUI student population was primarily, though not entirely, Catholic. His figures on the denominational organisation of the medical profession are statistical sectarianism in action.[55] Stafford Johnson's work was partly a response to the Protestant domination of small hospitals. Protestants would have been over-represented, numerically speaking, in the profession. One could argue that the medical profession was noted for the triumph of proximity over performance, a tendency not unusual in the professions at that time.

The entire saga should be seen in the context of the struggle to shape the institutional ideology of the emerging Irish Free State. As Mary E. Daly has noted in relation to the Hospital Sweepstakes: 'this was not the sole instance where the Catholic Church acted to prevent an expansion of social services that might upset the existing equilibrium between the state and the voluntary sector: during the 1930s proposals to extend access to post-primary schooling were successfully thwarted by the combined opposition of the Church and the Department of Finance.'[56] The Catholic Church's control of health and education was difficult to challenge.

The politics of children's health, 1928–39 105

Their opposition to new hospitals and schools which would not be under their control was fortified by the conservatism of state officials.

In February 1937 Lynn reported that an 'impasse over amalgamation had been reached'. However, undeterred, the medical committee suggested a scheme for a new hospital which would have 300 beds including 60 for a TB unit.[57] The hospital had received $6,488 from the United States in 1937, and the St Ultan's staff hoped to build their own hospital with a particular emphasis on children suffering from TB.[58] At the end of the 1930s, plans for the new hospital were 'considered in great detail' by the medical committee.[59] By then it was too late, the Second World War was about to begin and materials for building were scarce.

Lynn constantly hoped that her children's hospital would be built during the 1930s and '40s. However, it was not until after her death that a large children's hospital was opened. All of this turmoil exhausted but did not embitter Lynn. She was wary of Barry and when a new hospital, essentially an enlarged St Ultan's, without Harcourt Street, was mooted by Barry, she asked herself, 'what's she up to now?'[60] Later she referred to the 'Barry clique'.[61] It is to her credit that she regained her friendship with Alice Barry, but she never saw her hospital on the banks of the canal or Charlemont Street. It was not gender, but religion, which decided the fate of these energetic women and their children's hospital. Clearly, ecclesiastical might, not right, prevailed. Undeterred, the St Ultan's Utility Society sought to provide affordable accommodation. In some senses they were part of the slum clearances of this period, as local and national government sought to improve housing. Fahey has argued that the Fianna Fáil government put the housing of the urban poor at the centre of social policy. Slum clearance and the development of suburbs like Crumlin was, he suggests, 'one of the great social achievements of the day.[62] However, there were still housing problems for many and Lynn's work brought her into daily contact with those who lived in louse-ridden homes. Her surgery was 'crowded by the poor and needy'.[63]

DR MARIA MONTESSORI

Despite the frustrations of the 1930s, there were some celebrations. Lynn was an admirer of Dr Maria Montessori and her interest in education was furthered in 1934, when Dr Montessori (the first female physician in Italy) visited St Ultan's. Lynn thought the Italian doctor was 'beautiful' and gracious'.[64] Montessori was noted for advocating a child-centred approach to education. This view did not meet with the approval of Dr Timothy Corcoran, Professor of Education at UCD, who devoted several articles in *Irish Monthly* to Montessori education. He described it as 'braggart blasphemy'.[65] The amount of photographs devoted to young patients in the St Ultan's archives is striking. Unusually, they give only the names of the children, not the staff. The Montessori method is child-centred education, and St Ultan's offered child-centred medicine. Eventually, a Montessori school was established in St Ultan's. Many years later, Nancy Jordan, the St Ultan's Montessori teacher, was asked to speak at an International Montessori Congress in London about her work in St Ultan's.[66]

Like many middle-class reformers, Lynn had particular views on how others should behave. The children who lived near St Ultan's were in need of control, Lynn believed. 'We must try to reform the children in flats.'[67] She even suggested that some women one might expect to be careless were concerned about their children. 'The number of young flappers and "fiberty jiberty ones" that turn into excellent mothers is most surprising. There is a great love for babies.'[68] There was also a sense that women needed to nourished as they bore the future citizens of the nation. In 1938, Trinity scientist William Fearon wrote about the national problem of nutrition. During pregnancy, he argued, the 'maternal organism is bearing a double burden, often amid very unfavourable circumstances, and the effects of malnutrition during these critical periods are doubly unfortunate in that they effect the health of two individuals'.[69] Women were worthy of consideration because their health affected the vitality of future citizens. Furthermore, concerns about Ireland's declining population fuelled an increasing focus on nutrition which led to the great public health developments of the 1940s, including the introduction of the children's allowances in

1944. Unfortunately St Ultan's could only offer the equivalent of band aid when radical surgery was required.

NATIONAL AND INTERNATIONAL POLITICS

While Lynn's career was focused on medical care, she did not lose sight of her republican and socialist principles. In both politics and medicine, attempts to improve the lives of others were often halted because of the fear of socialism. A discussion of school meals was frustrating since providing meals to all was seen as interfering with family life. 'It is terrible that clergy hold it up', Lynn complained. However, it was not just certain clergymen who were wary of state involvement in family matters. Dr James McPolin, County Medical Officer for Limerick between 1930 and 1954, did not want to vaccinate children against smallpox. Diarmaid Ferriter suggests that his 'absolutist ideology' was a threat to the health of children.[70] These medical Richelieus were frequently in positions of power. Conservative beliefs were a reaction to the communism of the Soviet Union, where, Lynn mistakenly believed, socialism was 'succeeding wonderfully'.[71] Lynn, like many socialist intellectuals, was incredibly naive about the reality of life in the Soviet Union.[72] She saw communism as a form of Christianity.[73] The justice of all families receiving a fair wage was 'pure Bolshevism' and she linked this with the biblical parable of the labourers in the vineyard.[74] In essence, Lynn was a religious Bolshevik. She believed that the early Christians were 'all Communists'.[75] This commitment to communism was also allied to her anti-imperialism and she revelled in the success of Gandhi and the anti-imperialists in India. Their struggle against the British Empire mirrored Ireland's difficulties two decades earlier: 'tactics just like here, they won't let prisoners be visited'.[76] Lynn could also be humorous about imperialism. At the commemoration of the First World War, a 'poppy wearer at anti-Imperial meeting asked for police protection & the bobby put the poppy in his pocket saying he w[ou]ld be safe then'.[77]

Initially, Lynn had great hopes for the newly-elected Fianna Fáil government in 1932. She thought they would take a greater interest in socio-economic affairs. She wanted proper schemes for child welfare and improved housing conditions. Lynn gushed that the government had done great work in a single year.[78] Admittedly there were moves to improve antenatal care, particularly in Dublin where infant mortality was particularly high. 'By 1933, the antenatal clinics in all three of the Dublin maternity hospitals were co-ordinated with the county borough maternity and child welfare scheme, and subsidised by Dublin Corporation.'[79] However, her attitude gradually changed. The much-hated Conditions of Employment Bill of 1935 roused her. It sought to restrict the working hours of women. 'This regulation of conditions of work bill terrible, will deprive women fr. working. Where is 1916 Republican Proclamation.' Ffrench-Mullen shared her anger and wrote to the press regarding the 'injustice' of the bill.[80] Lynn described Lemass, the author of the bill, as 'antediluvian'.[81] Revealingly, in the Dáil, Lemass claimed that the legislation was 'not to secure employment for men now unemployed but to arrest any tendency to increasing female for male labour.'[82] It is not surprising that Lynn believed that 'the men were quite willing that we shld share dangers of war but now withhold fruits of it'.[83] There would be 'no Freedom' without women.[84] Yet, the Conditions of Employment Bill became an Act in 1936. Women had very little overt political power. Economics, as well as the ideological decision to employ men rather than women, dictated government policy. She even compared Fianna Fáil's actions with the ill treatment of the French Jew, Dreyfus. 'The trial reminded us so much of trials here where anything damning to Govt. promptly suppressed.'[85] Unfortunately, Ireland had no Emile Zola to expose injustices. By the end of the 1930s, Lynn thought that the government 'denied all they stood for before they were in power'.[86]

As well as becoming disillusioned with democratically elected governments, Lynn also despaired of her former republican friends. The Irish Republican Army were 'so self centred they would ruin Ireland to assert themselves'.[87] Later in 1933 she attended a Sinn Féin meeting but it 'was as futile as any before & degenerated into a squabble betwn. S.F. & the I.R.A. members present. Waste of time to go.'[88] She thought that the IRA had 'fallen far fr. 1916 ideals, alas they are just freebooters now, on the make'.[89]

Despite her disdain for republicans, she was concerned, as in the 1920s, about the ill treatment of republican prisoners. She thought that Fianna Fáil was 'worse than Cosgrave' (the leader of the opposition) in its treatment of political prisoners.[90] However, her attitude seemed to have changed by the end of the 1930s when she described the IRA as 'great lads [who] never shirk danger for Ireland's sake.'[91] It is not surprising, then, that Lynn should focus her considerable energies on medicine rather than politics.

Lynn was also painfully aware of international developments. As early as 1933 she thought that Germany was becoming 'more & more intolerant. It sounds fearful.'[92] Some months later she observed that 'Hitler has commanded clergy to throw out all Jews but D.V. some pastors won't have this unXtianity.'[93] She sensed that, as in the First World War, citizens would become cannon fodder. Her response was typical: 'Women must unite, why had they to rear children for gun fodder? Fascism unmasked. Germans work in Labour camp for keep, under military condit[ions] & they call it "employment."'[94] In 1938 she referred to the pogrom of 'poor, poor jews' in Germany.[95] Yet she remained totally unaware of similar injustices in the Soviet Union, where she believed, or convinced herself, that no one 'was hungry or out of work'![96] Lynn was under no illusions about Benito Mussolini, whom she described as 'awfully despotic'.[97] She remained resolutely anti-English throughout the 1930s and likened England to a 'poor mangey old lion!'[98] Not surprisingly, Lynn supported the republican side in the Spanish Civil War. As ever, her concern was for the rank and file, even if she did not share their ideology. General Eoin O'Duffy supported Franco; while his troops were having a 'horrid time in trenches', he was 'living in luxury'.[99] By 1939, when so many were fleeing Europe, and Ireland was reluctant to accept refugees, she moaned, 'poor homeless wanderers & that is how Christian!!! countries treat them. Oh! that we had more Faith.'[100] Later she was asked by Bethel Solomons, the Master of the Rotunda, to take refugee Jewish nurses at St Ultan's, which she was glad to do.[101]

1937 CONSTITUTION

After the demands of medical politics, Lynn was to be immersed briefly in national politics with the passage of the 1937 Constitution through the Irish parliament. Lynn thought the Constitution was 'reactionary'.[102] Through the Fianna Fáil organ, the *Irish Press*, de Valera endured the slings and arrows of outraged feminists. Many feminists were irritated by the proposed attempts to place women firmly in the home and deny them a public role. In June 1937 Lynn attended an anti-Constitution meeting at the Mansion House, ironically, the scene of much of her political activity two decades earlier. She proposed that the retention of the offending articles posed a 'menace' to the 'economic position of women'. Furthermore, she argued that 'were it not for working women many families would starve. There would have been no Easter Week, but for the women, but the position secured then had gradually been infringed upon since. The present man-ruled world was a sorry place, and would not be improved unless it were run by men and women on terms of equality.' Lynn's resolution was 'carried amid applause.'[103] Unwisely, and inaccurately, the *Irish Press* sneered at the 'feminine alarms'. The paper suggested that the 'learned ladies, whose zeal in the national cause has in many cases been hitherto conspicuous by its absence were not qualified to comment on the constitution'.[104] This was too much for Lynn whose response appeared two days later. First of all she alluded to women who had given sterling service in 1916 and thereafter, but she also castigated the present Fianna Fáil government by questioning its republican qualifications. 'The writer of the leader speaks as if zeal for the national cause and zeal for the Fianna Fáil party were synonymous terms.' However, 'we republicans do not support the present government which is merely the successor of the Cumann na nGaedheal government', she asserted. No doubt *Irish Press* readers appreciated that comparison! Finally, she pointed out that 'women of every political affiliation' were in the Mansion House and they were involved in 'some aspect of the women's struggle for freedom during the last twenty years'.[105] While some of the offending phrases, such as the reference to women's 'inadequate strength', were removed, most of the protests came to naught. The constitution was passed by a narrow majority. Lynn saw Fianna Fáil as simply an extension of Cumann na nGaedheal. As for her former friend, de Valera, he was 'still wanting an Irish Republic!! What folly, but really he is just Fianna Fáil, no better.'[106] Her comments on the death of Tim Healy are equally venomous: 'so passes the man who sold Ireland time & time again'.[107] Clearly Lynn had become disillusioned with national politics. Sinn Féin, the political party she had represented, was 'rotten'.[108] She stayed in contact with her Irish Citizen Army friends, however. In 1937 she became President of the Old ICA Association.[109]

SOCIAL LIFE

From the 1920s, Lynn was a regular visitor to Glenmalure in County Wicklow. Her good friend Susie Nugent was from Wicklow, and Lynn enjoyed her annual summer break in the beautiful surroundings of this valley. The cottage where she stayed had originally belonged to Maud Gonne MacBride who sold it to James Whelan in 1928. Lynn became the owner in 1937.[110] This was her spiritual home and a welcome relief from the tensions of her busy life in Dublin. Both literally and metaphorically, Lynn let her hair down in Glenmalure. Andrée Sheehy Skeffington, Hanna's granddaughter, suggested that Lynn's 'belief in the curative properties of fresh air and drinks of cold water were legendary in the family circle. She practised what she preached, as anyone could judge when visiting her cottage retreat at the end of the lonely Glenmalure Valley . . . To see her walking uphill barefoot to milk the goat, or collecting water from a mountain stream, was a source of wonder to visitors from abroad.'[111] Despite Lynn's antipathy to de Valera, Dorothy Macardle wrote her eulogy on the Irish Republic, which she dedicated to de Valera, in the Glenmalure cottage.

Lynn's holidays were not confined to Ireland. She also travelled extensively and managed to combine professional activities with pleasure. While in Zurich in 1929, she admired the children's hospitals and the wonderful sights. However cosmopolitan in her medical perspectives, she retained her political partisanship and complained that there were 'too many Union Jacks'.[112] Lynn returned two years later to attend a Hospitals' Congress. Undoubtedly, her fluency in German was a big advantage. On her return she reported to the St Ultan's medical committee on various new treatments.[113] In 1933 she visited the Hospitals Congress' in Belgium.[114]

Michael Scott, the famous architect, designed a balcony outside Lynn's bedroom so that she could sleep outdoors. Even during the winter months she enjoyed the bracing fresh air provided by her nocturnal outdoor activity. This sometimes reached incredible lengths. One January she mentioned sleeping 'v. well on balcony & waked to find it had frozen fairly hard'.[115] Lynn also enjoyed her garden and her gramophone and the latter was sometimes brought to Wicklow. Gardening provided a therapeutic outlet for Lynn and she admitted to 'longing to garden'.[116]

Lynn also enjoyed the 'clever' and 'amusing' comic talents of Jimmy O'Dea and looked forward to his Christmas pantomime.[117] She was in good health and was a sturdy 133 pounds (fifty-eight kilograms). At the sprightly age of 55 she 'tobogganed with the girls on ladder, gt. fun.'[118] While staying with Muriel she 'did gymnastics' and was 'more limber' than her younger sister.[119] Lynn was also blessed with great endurance and walked fifteen miles one summer's day while in her late fifties.[120]

Ardbraccan too provided annual sustenance every September. It even attracted American visitors. Mrs Hurley of Boston, who was 'truly Gaelic in every way', attended the outing in 1929.[121] After one outing in Ardbraccan, Lynn thanked God for the 'Peace & the cows & the fields'.[122] Furthermore, Lynn loved old Irish stories. She told the folklorist Bríd Mahon folktales which she had heard 'from the lips of Lady Gregory', one of the founders of the Abbey Theatre.[123]

Lynn's elder sister Nan died from TB in Grangegorman Asylum in September 1931, so Muriel was the only sibling still in Ireland. Despite their divergent political perspectives, Lynn regularly visited Muriel in Warrenpoint.[124] Her brother John returned to Ireland in 1932 from New York and stayed with Lynn, much to her delight. He made himself useful by doing odd jobs around the house, where his skills as an engineer were valued. Later he returned to his family in Australia after the death of his wife Anna.[125]

Lynn, then, despite her many activities, had an active social life. However, if ffrench-Mullen was away then Lynn was 'lonely'.[126] Ffrench-Mullen frequently attended spas abroad in order to improve her rheumatism. She received a salary from St Ultan's and, on occasion, the hospital funded her trips. Lynn's income, in retrospect, does not seem that impressive, given that she was an experienced medical practitioner. She complained that she had to pay £60 a year in income tax. Tax was five shillings in the pound, or 25 per cent; this would suggest an income of £240. It was certainly far above the salary of most people, with teachers earning about £150 per annum. Local folklore in Rathmines suggested that she did not charge fees from many of her patients. However, she admitted that she had to curtail her expenditure.[127] She always had a maid, even if her attitude was, on occasion, authoritarian. 'Mary gave notice at b.[reak]fast because I asked her to say please & not order me.'[128] Clearly, Lynn was the one giving the orders. Mary stayed on so they must have settled their differences.

CONCLUSION

At the 1936 Annual General Meeting of St Ultan's, the nationalist historian Dorothy Macardle suggested that the 'infant appealed to all, it had no politics'.[129] Nothing could have been further from the truth. Children's health was a contentious issue, particularly in the ideologically-divided 1930s. Lynn had to learn this uncomfortable reality. Her great love for children would count for little in the sectarian atmosphere of Irish medical politics. She argued that 'if a baby was to thrive in hospital it must not only receive the necessary care, it must be loved . . . Babies must be loved if they were to be cured'.[130] However, without adequate space these babies became part of the infant mortality statistics of the 1930s. Given that the hospital only had space for about fifty infants its impact was inevitably limited. Nonetheless, it was correct to suggest that infants appealed to all. Throughout this period St Ultan's continued to receive funding from the United States.

Politically Lynn was a failure, but in socio-medical terms St Ultan's was a partial success. The entire amalgamation episode shocked Lynn who was used to getting her own way in the hospital. At one stage she suggested that none of the physicians interviewed for a position at St Ultan's was suitable since 'some would boss me & that wouldn't do!' Worse, Lynn could be cruel toward her domestic staff: 'Molly turned up early & I dismissed her at once, she is too clever for me, I fear.' [131] Nonetheless, the staff at St Ultan's and at 9 Belgrave Road, provided services for others when it was badly needed.

Ultimately, whatever about her power at home or in St Ultan's, Lynn could not defy the power of the Catholic Church in the Irish Free State. McQuaid and his acolytes were successful. By 1939, plans for the 'Catholic Children's Hospital' were being discussed. However, this hospital, which was named Our Lady's Hospital for Sick Children, with the Catholic Archbishop of Dublin as manager, did not open until 1956. For many children, it was too late.

NOTES

1 The most incisive analysis is provided by Finola Kennedy, *Cottage to Crèche: Family Change in Ireland* (Dublin, 2001), pp. 150–206.
2 David Sheehy, private conversation, at the Dublin Diocesan Archives.
3 Diarmaid Ferriter, review of Finola Kennedy, *Cottage to Crèche: Family Change in Ireland*, in *The Economic and Social Review*, vol. 33, no. 2, summer/autumn, 2002, pp. 259–62, p. 261.
4 *Catholic Bulletin*, 2 Feb., 1931, vol. 21, no2, p. 143, quoted in Dermot Keogh, *The Vatican, the Bishops and Irish Politics, 1919–39* (Cambridge, 1986), p. 169.
5 Catholic ethics were a matter of considerable concern; see John H. Harty, 'The Church and Science' in *Irish Ecclesiastical Record*, vol. vii, Jan – June, 1900, pp. 158–71.
6 Dermot Keogh, *Twentieth-Century Ireland: Nation and State* (Dublin, 1994), p. 58.
7 Denis Boyle, *A History of Meath County Council, 1899–1999: A Century of Democracy in Meath* (Navan, 1999), p. 151; Margaret Ó hÓgartaigh, 'A medical apppointment in County Meath' in *Ríocht na Midhe: Records of the Meath Archaeological and Historical Society*, vol. xvii, 2006, pp. 266–70.
8 Jack White, *Minority Report: The Protestant Community in the Irish Republic* (Dublin, 1975), pp. 163–4.
9 Dr Gilmartin statement in Letitia Dunbar-Harrison file, Department of An Taoiseach S2547A, NAI; the case is discussed in a witty manner by J.J. Lee

The politics of children's health, 1928–39 115

in his *Ireland, 1912–1985* (Cambridge, 1989), pp. 161–68. Mary E. Daly has made clear the local dimension in the selection of candidates for local authority positions; see 'Local Appointments', in Mary E. Daly (ed.) *County and Town.:One Hundred Years of Local Government in Ireland* (Dublin, 2001), pp. 45–55.
10 Robert Collis, *To be a Pilgrim* (London, 1975), p. 76.
11 Alan Browne was told this as an undergraduate in Trinity College Dublin in the 1940s. He served as Master of the Rotunda between 1960 and 1966; his comment was made at the History Section Meeting of the Royal Academy of Medicine in Ireland, April 2000.
12 Interview with Dr Pearl Dunlevy, February 1996.
13 *Report of the Department of Local Government and Public Health, 1932–33*, p. 54. I am grateful to Dr Lindsey Earner Byrne for a copy of her paper '"In Respect of Motherhood": an Irish Catholic Social Service, 1930–1954', which was presented to the Irish Historical Society, November 1999.
14 St Ultan's Medical Committee, 25 April 1934, SUA.
15 St Ultan's Medical Committee, 10 October and 24 October 1934, SUA.
16 St Ultan's Medical Committee, 10 April 1935, SUA.
17 For a discussion of the development of the Hospitals' Sweepstakes, see Marie Coleman, 'The origins of the Irish Hospitals' Sweepstake', in *Irish Economic and Social History*, vol. xxix, 2002, pp. 40–56.
18 St Ultan's General Board, 20 Nov. 1930, SUA.
19 St Ultan's General Board, 30 May 1935, SUA.
20 St Ultan's General Board, 17 Jan. 1935, SUA.
21 Lindsay Earner-Byrne, 'In respect of motherhood': maternity policy and provision in Dublin city, 1922–1956' (Ph.D., UCD, 2001), p. 51.
22 St Ultan's General Board, 16 Jan, 1930, SUA.
23 Greta Jones, 'The Rockefeller and medical education in Ireland in the 1920s', in *Irish Historical Studies*, vol. xxx, no. 120, Nov. 1997, pp. 564–80.
24 Mary E. Daly, '"An Atmosphere of Sturdy Independence" : the State and the Dublin Hospitals in the 1930s Dublin Hospitals' in Elizabeth Malcolm and Greta Jones (eds), *Medicine, Disease and the State* (Cork, 1999) pp. 234–52, p. 238.
25 Coleman, 'Hospitals' Sweepstake', p. 51.
26 Evelyn Bolster, *Knights of Columbanus* (Dublin, 1974), p. 75. Stafford Johnson was the supreme knight between 1942 and 1948.
27 Aidan Lehane C.S.Sp., 'The Visitor', in *Studies*, winter, 1998, vol. 87, no. 348, pp. 392–95. I am grateful to Fr. Lehane who discussed his memories of McQuaid and Stafford Johnson's visits to Rockwell College, personal communication, 20 Dec. 2002. McQuaid and Stafford Johnson frequently holidayed together.
28 Stafford Johnson to Byrne, 31 Nov. 1931, Byrne Papers Box One: Lay Organisations, Dublin Diocesan Archives (hereafter DDA), cited in Earner-Byrne, '"In Respect of Motherhood": maternity policy and provision in Dublin city, 1922–1956', p. 74.
29 Perhaps some of Lea-Wilson's resentment towards St Ultan's stemmed from the fact that several of the St Ultan's doctors were clearly republican

in outlook. It was generally believed that Lea-Wilson's husband, Major Percival Lea-Wilson, was executed by republicans as a reprisal for his ill treatment of 1916 prisoners, in particular the elderly Tom Clarke, in Parnell Square after the 1916 Rising. She wrote to Dr Byrne about her colleagues in Harcourt Street, describing several of them as, 'C of I, f.m', that is, Church of Ireland, Free Mason. See Byrne Papers (Hospitals General), DDA. She was very aware of the denominational divisions in Irish medicine.
30 Finola Kennedy, personal conversation, 20 Dec. 2002.
31 LD, 3 and 4 Jan. 1935.
32 Davis Coakley, *Irish Masters of Medicine* (Dublin, 1992), pp. 325–6. Coakley believes that Dr Price 'was largely responsible for the elimination of childhood tuberculosis in Ireland', p. 326.
33 Collis, *To be a Pilgrim*, p. 71.
34 LD, 5 Jan. 1935.
35 LD, 17 Jan. 1935
36 LD, 24 Jan. 1935.
37 LD, 14 August 1935.
38 LD, 12 Nov. 1935.
39 LD 14 Nov. 1935.
40 St Ultan's Medical Committee, 20 Nov. 1935, SUA.
41 LD, 20 Nov. 1935
42 LD, 21 Nov. 1935.
43 LD, 28 Nov. 1935.
44 LD, 9 Dec. 1935.
45 LD, 20 Dec. 1935.
46 *Irish Times*, 16 Nov. 1935.
47 Response of Dr Byrne in Joint Hospitals File, SUA.
48 St Ultan's response in Joint Hospitals File, SUA.
49 Lynn to Byrne, 27 Jan. 1936, in Byrne Papers (Hospitals General), DDA.
49 McQuaid to Byrne 11 Dec 1936 Byrne Papers (Hospitals General), DDA.
50 Greta Jones, 'Marie Stopes in Ireland – The Mothers' Clinic in Belfast, 1936–47', in *Social History of Medicine*, vol. 5, no. 2, 1992, pp. 255–77, pp. 267–68.
51 John Cooney, *John Charles McQuaid: Ruler of Catholic Ireland* (Dublin, 1999).
52 McQuaid to Byrne, 11 Dec. 1936, Byrne Papers (Hospitals General), DDA.
53 LD, 13 Feb. 1936.
54 Medical Committee, 1 April 1936, SUA.
55 See Byrne Papers (Hospitals General) 1935–39, DDA, for Stafford Johnson's very careful analyses of the staffing in Dublin hospitals.
56 Daly, 'Dublin Hospitals' p. 250.
57 Medical Committee, 24 Feb. 1937, SUA.
58 St Ultan's General Board, 20 May 1937, SUA.
59 St Ultan's Medical Committee, 8 Feb. 1939, SUA.
60 LD, 4 Jan. 1937.
61 LD, 20 Oct. 1938.

62 Tony Fahey, 'Housing and Local Government' in Daly (ed.), *County and Town*, pp. 120–29, p. 123.
63 Seamus Ó Maitiú, *Rathmines Township, 1847–1930* (Dublin, 1997), p. 27. Such was the extent of urban squalor that Ireland still had louse-borne typhus in the 1940s, and was the last 'last country in western Europe' to be infected with typhus. James Deeny, *The End of an Epidemic: Essays in Irish Public Health, 1935–65* (Dublin, 1995), p. 53.
64 LD, 20 Jan. 1934.
65 Timothy Corcoran, 'Is the Montessori Method to be introduced into Irish Schools?' *Irish Monthly*, March 1924, pp. 118–24.
66 LD, 11 May 1951.
67 LD, 8 June 1935.
68 Newspaper cutting, 28 May 1942, ffrench-Mullen scrapbook.
69 William Fearon, 'The national problem of nutrition', in *Studies*, March 1938, vol. 27, p. 17.
70 Diarmaid Ferriter, 'Local Government, public health and welfare in twentieth-century Ireland', in Daly (ed.), *County and Town*, pp. 109–19, p. 116.
71 4 Dec. 1929.
72 LD, 20 Feb. 1930.
73 LD, 4 April 1930.
74 LD, 15 Sept. 1930.
75 LD, 19 Oct. 1931.
76 LD, 22 May 1930.
77 LD, 11 Nov. 1933.
78 LD, 24 Jan. 1934.
79 Earner-Byrne, '"In respect of motherhood": maternity policy and provision in Dublin city, 1922–1956' p. 52.
80 LD, 12 and 13 June 1935.
81 LD, 28 June 1935.
82 Dáil Debates, 17 May, 1917, cited in Mary E. Daly, *Industrial Development and Irish National Identity, 1922–39* (Dublin, 1992), p. 126.
83 LD, 8 Nov. 1935.
84 LD, 5 Dec. 1935.
85 LD, 22 March 1938.
86 LD, 16 Feb. 1939.
87 LD, 6 Sept. 1933.
88 LD, 23 Oct. 1933.
99 LD, 29 Nov. 1933.
90 LD, 21 July and 5 Sept. 1936.
91 LD, 30 May 1939.
92 LD, 19 June 1933.
93 LD, 14 Nov. 1933.
94 LD, 1 Sept. 1934.
95 LD, 11 Nov. 1938.
96 LD, 19 Sept. 1934.

97 LD, 18 May 1936.
98 LD, 11 June 1936.
99 LD, 26 May 1937.
100 LD, 2 April 1939.
101 LD, 6 May 1939.
102 LD, 13 May 1937.
103 *Irish Press*, 22 June 1937.
104 *Irish Press*, 23 June 1937.
105 *Irish Press*, 25 June 1937.
106 LD, 30 May 1930.
107 LD, 27 March 1931.
108 LD, 22 Sept. 1931.
109 LD, 6 Dec. 1937.
110 Information derived from Folio 2826, Co. Wicklow, in the Land Registry Offices, Dublin by Andrew O'Brien. I am very grateful for his generosity in sharing his great knowledge of County Wicklow with me.
111 Andrée Sheehy Skeffington, *Skeff: The Life of Owen Sheehy Skeffington, 1909–1970* (Dublin, 1991), p. 26.
112 LD 15 May 1929.
113 St Ultan's Medical Committee, 16 July 1931, SUA.
114 St Ultan's Medical Committee, 12 July 1933, SUA.
115 LD, 3 Jan. 1931.
116 LD, 11 March 1929. Lynn also played the gramophone to patients on the roof of St Ultan's, LD, 17 March 1937.
117 LD, 21 April 1928.
118 LD, 16 Feb. 1929.
119 LD, 16 August 1931.
120 LD, 6 May 1933.
121 LD, 1 Sept. 1929.
122 LD, 4 Sept. 1932.
123 Bríd Mahon, *While the Grass Grows: Memoirs of a Folklorist* (Cork, 1998), p. 150.
124 LD, 28 Sept. 1931.
125 LD, 28 Nov. 1937.
126 LD, 16 Sept. 1928.
127 LD, 11 Oct. 1932.
128 LD, 6 Feb. 1939.
129 St Ultan's General Committee, 28 May 1936, SUA.
130 St Ultan's General Committee, 27 May 1937, SUA.
131 LD, 3 Oct. 1930. Nellie was 'sulky & weepy', so Lynn decided to 'let her go', LD, 1 Dec. 1930. 'Molly' dismissed, LD, 20 May 1931.

CHAPTER FIVE

A servant of the nation, 1940–55

ONE MIGHT HAVE expected Lynn's life to show some slowing down as she reached her mid sixties in 1940. However, the last fifteen years of her life were filled with activity. She was kept busy nurturing Second World War refugees. Furthermore, the National BCG Centre was established at St Ultan's in 1949. Tuberculosis eradication, and the housing of the Dublin poor provided a sociomedical focus for Lynn. Throughout her career, she was concerned with illnesses which were exacerbated by socio-economic deprivation. The public health developments of the twentieth century made a career in medicine fulfilling, if frustrating. In some ways, this period saw the realisation of some of her aspirations.

Nonetheless, as in the 1930s, medical politics often impeded her work. The conflicts between Dr James Deeny, Chief Medical Officer at the Department of Local Government and Public Health, and later the Department of Health, and Dr Noël Browne, the Minister for Health, delayed the implementation of much-needed medical schemes. Both were active in social medicine but neither was noted for his humility, and they were to clash over the best method to eliminate TB.[1] These two dynamic and determined individuals clashed even before Browne became Minister for Health in 1948. Deeny argued that TB was spread by contagion and Browne took issue with him. These two confident men clashed in the Custom House,[2] where the Department of Health was based. Paradoxically they simultaneously drove and impeded the TB eradication campaign. Deeny, the son of a socially concerned Lurgan doctor was a student in the exclusive, Jesuit-run Clongowes College in the 1910s. Many years later he said that his education at Clongowes, 'gave me the notion of social responsibility and social care and it altered my whole life'.[3] However, he was a 'Catholic populist' who was very critical of inertia in medicine.[4] By the 1940s, the radicalisation of TB patients was underway under the energetic direction of Browne. He had personally suffered from the ravages of the disease and many of his family fell victim to TB. Patients and their families had become frustrated with the slow rate of change in the provision of services for the ill. Browne reflected and harnessed this frustration. Part of the politicisation and radicalisation of TB could be attributed to the poor rate of progress during the 1930s and early 1940s. Furthermore, sanatoria faced long waiting lists, and conditions in these institutions were often grim. This radicalised TB patients and their families.[5] In 1944 the Post Sanatorium League was established and it sought to support discharged TB patients. The League brought 'the issue of poverty and tuberculosis into the public spotlight'.[6] Lynn was to be part of the radicalisation of health care in the 1940s.

There were several lay Catholics whose views on Protestant involvement in medicine, mirrored, if not magnified, those of John Charles McQuaid. Dr James McPolin, the Medical Officer for Health in Limerick, and, significantly, an Ulster Catholic was, like McQuaid, resolute in his determination to avoid any hint of state medical aid. He had been working in the Mater in Belfast during the pogroms of the early 1920s, and this surely coloured his views.[7] Hence there was a desire to ensure that Catholics of the correct ideological mindset were placed in key positions. This would automatically have excluded Lynn. In 1942, John Duffy, acting joint honorary secretary of the Irish National Tuberculosis League, confided in McQuaid:

> To secure a preponderance of Catholic representation I have succeeded, as I had planned, in having the county branches of the League placed under the guidance of the County Medical Officers of Health, practically all of whom are Catholics, and many of them leading Catholic Actionists.

McQuaid's marginalia makes clear his support: 'I approve and assure you in advance of support of Cath. Social Service Conference.'[8] Clearly professional rivalries, as well as concerns regarding the provision of care for children, played their part. Jones has referred to the 'Catholicisation of Peamount' in the 1940s.[9] Given Peamount's origins as a TB sanatorium established by the WNHA, clearly there were changes in medicine which reflected changes in society. The Catholicisation of medicine affected Lynn and her colleagues. Dorothy Price was the acting joint secretary of the Anti-Tuberculosis League with John Duffy. Medical scholars like Price wanted to focus on the medical aspects of TB, but they were overwhelmed by the activities of the medical politicians. Price's friend Dr J.M. O'Donovan, Professor of Medicine at UCC, attended a Red Cross meeting in 1944 and asked Price to 'exert any pressure' to aid the prevention of TB.[10] His frustration with the activities of the Red Cross is all too clear:

> I am glad you take the same view as I do about joining the Red Cross; in this town [Cork] at least it is quite obviously in political hands, and I feel extremely uncomfortable in the company of those who are running it. Of course one should not let this feeling interfere with good work, but there is an insincerity about the whole set-up which would defeat any useful co-operation on my part, and, like you, I feel happier in doing my own clinical work and such preventive work as I can personally undertake or inspire. After all, I consider that by teaching a batch of students each year how to face the problem in their individual practices afterwards, I am doing at least as much good as sitting around the table with a motley crew who are so vocal but, not very co-operative.[11]

These political issues, as in the 1930s, would stall the provision of a clear plan for the elimination of TB. Furthermore, there were major socio-medical issues, such as the poor state of housing which contributed to the spread of TB. Lynn, after her experiences in the 1930s with Byrne, McQuaid's predecessor, should have been prepared for the political difficulties surrounding the provision of child health facilities. There were particular concerns in the 1940s that state involvement would lead to socialism or even communism. When Dr Stafford Johnson, who was so active in the plans for a Catholic children's hospital, became Supreme Knight in the Knights of Columbanus, the Beveridge Plan was on the agenda.

There were fears that improved medical provision and welfare in Britain would expose Irish inadequacies. Stafford Johnson believed the Beveridge was 'a means through which an unacceptable solution would be foisted on the country by England and America . . . An integrally Catholic State is the one and only solution'.[12] McQuaid became a member of the Knights in 1947. Even more worryingly, Stafford Johnson wished to establish ' a virile legal unit in Ely House which would assist in drafting suitable legislation on problems for presentation to the responsible minister'. Evelyn Bolster, the historian of the Knights of Columbanus, and a member of the Sisters of Mercy, suggested, in an illuminating aside, that Stafford Johnson was refering to 'the incompatibility of ecclesiastical and civil law on some issues'.[13] Secular authorities were seen as unsound on certain matters. As with the development of a children's hospital, McQuaid ensured that when the TB preventorium at Ballyroan was being built the religious orders would provide the nursing.[14] On one hand this suited the state, since religious orders had a long tradition of providing social services. However, secular women lost out, in particular, those, like Lynn, who sought an independent role in the provision of childcare.

As national politics was radicalised in the late 1940s with the election of the first inter-party government after sixteen years of Fianna Fáil, Lynn was forced to work with visionary and demanding medical politicians such as Browne. Furthermore, her colleague Dr Dorothy Price had, by this stage, an international reputation as an expert on childhood TB.[15] The politicisation of the disease had implications for the delivery of medical services. The omnipotent Catholic Archbishop, McQuaid, took a very dim view of many Protestant doctors. He was assiduous in ensuring that Catholic doctors treated Catholic patients. Furthermore, he wanted his own carefully selected candidates to infiltrate and dominate the national Anti-Tuberculosis League which had been established by the medical profession in 1942. McQuaid wanted all members of the League to be part of the Irish Red Cross because it reflected the aspirations of Catholic social activists such as his friend Judge Conor Maguire. These attempts to pack medical committees with carefully selected candidates were to frustrate the work of Lynn and others who sought to improve people's lives.

The beginning of the 1940s saw Lynn's life unchanged in so many respects. As ever she was concerned about her patients and the treatment of the poor in an impoverished economy. Even when her home was raided for arms she was rather nostalgic as it was 'quite like old times.'[16] She still visited Glenmalure during the summer with her canine companion, the beloved Bran. Lynn also spent quite a lot of time caring for the increasingly wayward Helena (Emer) Molony.

'THE EMERGENCY'

Ireland was officially neutral during the Second World War and this period was known euphemistically as 'the Emergency'. With rationing and censorship, Ireland was cut off from many of the events of the 1940s. At this time Lynn was left with greater familial responsibilities. The death of her aunt, Florence Wynne, in September 1941 severed yet another link with Lynn's mother. Lynn felt 'really lost & lonely' without Florence.[17] However, Lynn remained close to her Wynne relatives and had a special affection for William (Billy) Wynne, who became a Church of Ireland clergyman. Later in 1941 she lost her good friend and long-time member of the St Ultan's board, Mary Cosgrave. Lynn was very active on the memorial committee for Cosgrave. Characteristically though, she did not stay long at a dance in the Mansion House for the Cosgrave Memorial as she feared ffrench-Mullen would want her.[18] Ffrench-Mullen's health was in decline and Lynn fretted over her.

Like many others during the war, Lynn grew her own vegetables.[19] She saw that children died from 'malnutrition', but it was 'really starvation & neglect'.[20] The war posed particular difficulties for the urban poor. There were 29 dispensary districts in the Dublin metropolitan area which were served by 43 doctors, but they were expected to cater for 6,220 people.[21] However, one unexpected side effect of the war was the increasing awareness of the extent of social distress.[22] The demand for Irish labour in war-torn Britain escalated. Delousing of future emigrants made such an impression on T.J. McElligott, the parsimonious secretary of the

Department of Finance, that he uncharacteristically gave funding for public health initiatives. While the average consumption of calories in Ireland was considerably higher than most European countries,[23] admittedly while they endured a destructive war, the poor living standards and inadequate diet endured by the urban poor was a focus for several commentators. In 1943 Dr Charles Clancy Gore presented a report to the Statistical and Social Inquiry Society of Ireland on the nutritional standards of Dublin working-class families. Of the 684 persons surveyed, 459 people, or more than two-thirds, were at a subsistence level. More revealingly, the Clancy Gore report revealed that women were inclined to go without in times of extreme need. In the UK, Margaret Mitchell noticed that the 'more striking effects of deprivation on maternal rather than infant mortality is due to the fact that the poor nutrition of a pregnant woman is likely to exact a greater toll on her health, and in severe cases her life, than it is on her infant's. In the 1930s it was four times more dangerous to bear a child than to work in a coal mine.'[24] The McCourt-like existence endured by many of the urban and rural poor ensured that preventing disease was a particular problem.[25] These enormous difficulties had to be surmounted. As one writer suggested in *The Journal of the Medical Association of Éire*, 'to preach health to the underfed or overcrowded is a hypocrisy'.[26] Hence Lynn was not unique in her concern for the welfare of others. Dr James Deeny, then a general practitioner in Lurgan, had also conducted research on malnutrition. Lynn was impressed by his talk on infant mortality to the Statistical and Social Inquiry Society of Ireland, which was subsequently published.[27] It is noticeable that there was increasing concern about the links between malnutrition and illness. Clearly Lynn was part of a generation of social activists who sought, occasionally in diametrically different ways, to ameliorate the lives of others. Problematically, when the United Kingdom was contemplating the introduction of the Welfare State in the aftermath of the Beveridge report, ideological battles were being fought over the best method of improving social services. These debates over welfare would spill over into ideological and denominational battles.

Lynn faced the loss of her great friend Madeleine ffrench-Mullen in May 1944. 'My darling M' died peacefully.[28] Not surprisingly Lynn was 'so lonely for dearest MffM'.[29] The loss of her long-time friend only added to Lynn's travails. For the remaining decade of her life Lynn continually invoked the memory of her friend, the 'dear one'. When difficulties arose at St Ultan's, Lynn suggested that ffrench-Mullen would have dealt with them tactfully and efficiently.

However difficult things were, and however lonely Lynn felt, she was always aware of the sufferings of others. The war posed particular problems for those in institutions. Lynn met Dr Anna McCabe, medical inspector of industrial schools, who thought the diet available was 'often insufficient'.[30] McCabe also admitted to being 'appalled' at the deprivation endured in these schools.[31] Lynn's work on a range of bodies from the Child Health Council to St Ultan's would never fully come to grips with the problems facing child welfare activists. Part of the difficulty lay with the training of medical professionals. Lynn noted that a postgraduate course ignored paediatrics although it was 'a good half of Medicine & the most important half'.[32] Clearly, the malnutrition, or, more precisely, semi-starvation, endured by the urban and rural poor in these years was a concern. McQuaid had established the Catholic Social Service Conference in 1941 in order to co-ordinate and Catholicise various social services. It provided over a quarter of a million meals per month during the war years.[33] However, McQuaid encouraged 'Catholic supremacy' whereas, in the past, there had been some overlap between Catholic and Protestant social services.[34] Despite impressive work on behalf of the needy, by the end of the 1940s Ireland still had one of the highest maternal and infant mortality rates in western Europe.[35]

The war was not all doom and gloom. Lynn's interest in Irish was boosted when a new church on Adelaide Road was opened for Irish services in January 1945. Much to her delight it 'was packed & nearly all young'.[36] The following month, she noted that it was the 40th anniversary of Irish services on St Patrick's Day.[37] Dr Dónal Caird, later Church of Ireland Archbishop of Dublin, had a distinctive memory of Lynn's work for Cumann Gaelach na hEaglaise:

A small old lady, who wore pince-nez spectacles and who always arrived on an ancient bicycle wearing rather incongruously a long fur coat in the winter, which she managed miraculously to keep out of the spokes of the moving wheels, I learnt to be the famous Dr Kathleen Lynn . . . She looked so mild and spoke so gently that it was hard to believe that less than thirty years previously she had taken part in the Rebellion of 1916 . . . She looked as though she had been involved in nothing more exciting in her life than a spelling bee, as would have become the daughter of an archdeacon of the Church of Ireland from the Diocese of Tuam, which she was. She was an effective champion of Dublin's poor, a staunch and unyielding Republican, and a devout member of the Church of Ireland. She was very keen to develop the social side of life for those interested in Irish, so she arranged mid-week céilithe during the winter to attract young people into the language movement.[38]

Caird also remembered Lynn with her friend Lil Nic Dhonnchadha, the principal at Coláiste Móibhí, an All-Irish Preparatory College for Protestants, establishing the K Club for young people on Molesworth Street in Dublin. Lynn had helped to paint the wall white and the chairs red.[39] The war years were difficult, but they were not completely joyless.

ST ULTAN'S

Despite the adverse conditions endured by many Lynn remained resolute in her medical views. She had always been against comforters, as children could pick up infections from them and she admitted to losing her temper with a patient over comforters.[40] Lynn wanted to prevent the spread of infection. Her attitude was not unique. Dr Elizabeth Bell's comments on artificial feeding constituted 'thinly veiled disapproval', as she believed that this kind of feeding facilitated infections.[41] Lynn declared that the 'great object of the hospital was to instruct mothers how to bring up their children so that illness might be avoided'.[42] Yet she did not always reign supreme over staff. On one occasion, Lynn complained that the matron, Nan Dougan, was 'unreasonable as usual'.[43] Lynn could be quite cutting about her colleagues. She once noted that at the St Ultan's board there was 'no one of intelligence there but Dr O'Doherty'.[44] Despite her obvious concern for others, she still remained an unyielding employer. 'In Teac [St Ultan's] all maids are leaving, perhaps just as well, they are out of hand & always telling one another that this & that is not their work. The present day is hard on employers.'[45] This was a middle-class concern and Lynn was articulating the views of those who saw their role as the guardians of the working class.

Like Lynn, John Charles McQuaid was concerned about deprivation, and Lynn praised his asceticism. He 'had banquet of scrambled eggs & tea on evg. of the Consecration. He gives all to poor, 3,000 bags [of] coal in Xmas week.'[46] Little did she realise that the large children's hospital at Crumlin was part of McQuaid's fiefdom. By 1941 she noticed that the 'new Crumlin Hosp. for children is going ahead to blot us out!!'[47] Before long she realised that McQuaid was focused on Catholic control. 'I fear Abp. McQuaid is following in steps of predecessor forbids secret societies & education in any but R.C. schools & colleges.'[48] She also suggested that he 'fears any but R.Cs doing any social work'.[49] When the tragic fire at a Poor Clare Orphanage in Cavan Town in 1943 led to the deaths of thirty-five orphans and a cook, Lynn perceptively suggested that 'nuns will get away with anything but it shouldn't be & the reaction will be all the worse later & so many nuns are so really good'.[50] A tribunal exonerated the nuns and local government despite the patently inadequate fire prevention measures. However, Lynn was not entirely consistent in her attitudes. Catholic Bishop Dignan of Clonfert suggested a scheme for medical services but Lynn was critical, as she thought it 'seems so much as if the R.C. Church wants to run all Social Service as well as education. God grant a way out for us all.'[51] When the Minister for Local Government and Public Health, Sean MacEntee, criticised the Dignan plan, Lynn thought it was 'marvellous that anyone shld. reprimand the "Church"'.[52] Ironically, Dignan had a genuine concern for social welfare. Adrian Kelly has argued that it suited politicians to quote ecclesiastics when their views chimed with the economic requirements of the emerging state. However, when there were calls for children's allowances by the likes of Dr Cornelius

Lucey (Catholic Bishop of Cork, who was not noted for his *joie de vivre*, hence the nickname Cranky Con) then episcopal suggestions were ignored.[53] Likewise, Dignan was sidelined because his suggestions would have upset the delicate balance between the government and institutional Catholicism.

Lynn bemoaned the waste of money and the war's effect on the poor: '11 million can be spent a day on war, but for betterment of poor? No money at all for that.'[54] There were some bright lights on the horizon, however. Dr Dorothy Price was an expert on childhood tuberculosis and she had worked with Scott on the new TB extension at St Ultan's.[55] When Price's book on childhood TB was published in 1942, Lynn suggested that Price was 'great' for St Ultan's.[56] Price's work was essential since there were concerns about the connections between TB, ill health and malnutrition amongst the general population, as well as particular concerns about children. The feeding of schoolchildren was a contentious issue, yet the service was badly needed. Lynn reported that TCD and UCD were feeding 800 schoolchildren daily.[57] Lynn was all too aware of the need for social welfare. At St Ultan's in December 1942 she saw a child 'who has no clothes, 11 in family & £1.12.0 [£1.60] a week for everything'.[58] Lynn was also made aware of the disadvantages of running a female-dominated hospital. She was told to 'get into [the] graces' of the Local Government Department by having men on the St Ultan's board.[59] Mr McEvoy, President of the Federation of Irish Industries, and Stephen McGloughlin, a businessman, were co-opted on to the board.[60]

Conditions for those without material resources remained grim. During the harsh winter of 1946–47 Lynn bemoaned the spate of dying infants in St Ultan's. Tellingly she noted that there were 'no fires in poor houses'.[61] The winter had been so severe that even Lynn admitted it was 'ages' since she had slept on the balcony.[62]

NATIONAL POLITICS

Throughout the 1940s Lynn remained resolutely anti-government. 'Hear Med. Union v. up in arms agst. govt. re inaction in building schemes & general discourtesy & belittling of the Profession wh. comes fr. govt.'s crass ignorance.'[63] The lack of resources to improve the lives of ordinary people was frustrating but this combined with Lynn's disdain for Fianna Fáil. Later she referred to more 'autocratic actions of Govt. Talk about Hitler!'[64] Lynn also blamed the government's 'injustice & incompetence' for the poor regulation of much-needed fuel.[65] When the government adopted a hard-line attitude towards political prisoners, Lynn said that a 'kind of off with their heads regime [was] instituted.'[66] At the end of the war and, in a rare note of praise for de Valera, Lynn thought his celebrated response to Churchill was 'v. restrained & dignified'.[67] In general though, she was to remain critical of de Valera's Fianna Fáil government.

Lynn was an obvious magnet for republicans. Like many others, even those who did not share her republican views, she enjoyed the broadcasts of Lord Haw Haw, William Joyce, the Nazi propagandist. She did not enjoy pomp and circumstance, however. When Sean T. O'Kelly became Ireland's second president, she suggested, with a mixture of snobbery and compassion, that it was 'all in such bad taste for Plebians like him & Phyllis Ryan, perhaps she'll want coronet next & then money squandered on that & Europe starves. Horrible.'[68]

In 1947 Sinn Féin attempted to organise the funds which had been collected two decades before. Lynn was not impressed with de Valera's activities. 'Dev. absolutely unashamed of his bill to seize Sinn Féin funds, setting up Comt. to decide appointed by him.'[69] De Valera admitted in the Dáil in 1947 that Lynn and himself were the only survivors of the officer board of the Sinn Féin executive which had 'control of the organisation after the February Árd Fheis of 1922.'[70] Not surprisingly, Lynn was asked to give evidence at the Sinn Féin funds tribunal. However, Lynn claimed that when two young men asked her to become involved in the revival of Sinn Féin in 1949, she 'knew nothing now of politics one way or another'.[71]

While Lynn had become disillusioned with national politics, she still looked back with pride to earlier patriots. For the sesquicentenary of the 1798 Rebellion in 1948, she took part in a Dublin procession which celebrated the event. 'Started for '98

Procession, such crowds, had to take bus to Terenure to get back, it only went to Harcourt St, found Citizen Army & walked at head of our 1916 Red X. It was moving to see people I hadn't seen in years . . . we old ones were so glad to do it & many children there.'[72] Lynn also loaned her picture of Bishop Young, Wolfe Tone's tutor at Trinity, to the National Museum.[73] She heard a sermon at a 1798 commemoration service which suggested that all the prophets were revolutionaries.[74] This gave her sustenance as she saw a spiritual element in the fight for Irish independence. Fianna Fáil eventually lost power in 1948 but after three years of a coalition government they returned to the Dáil. Lynn remained unimpressed. 'Dev. has all his old crowd back & an inept lot they are except Lemass.'[75]

INTERNATIONAL POLITICS

Despite Lynn's obvious reservations about Hitler throughout the 1930s, she delighted in German victories. Perhaps this can be explained by her obsessional hatred for Britain. Early in June 1940, when the German army was only twenty miles from Paris she gushed, 'how wonderful they are!'[76] More wittily, she suggested that the 'British are v. pious for it is always on Retreat'.[77] Despite Lynn's obvious glee at the difficulties faced by the Allies, she continually hoped and prayed for peace. More inexplicably, she became very critical of Russia and favoured Germany. Her former support for Russia waned as they were 'grabbing all they can lay hold of.'[78] Given her clear support for communism, this political turnabout can only be explained by her desire to see Britain isolated. Clearly she supported the Axis and not the Allies. This is reflected in her comments on Japan which she described as 'wonderful'.[79] Lynn also hoped that Hitler would 'succeed'.[80] Incredibly, she thought that a speech made by Hitler in October 1942 was 'determined & dignified' and 'not ranting'.[81] Even more disconcerting are Lynn's views on Jews. In the midst of the war she declared, 'everything here acting into Jewish hands, true, alas!'[82] She even suggested that those who favoured Jewish business ensured that the 'Hitlers retaliate & one knows why. We shld strive

A servant of the nation, 1943 131

& strive to convert the Jews.'[83] These views were not uncommon amongst Christians, yet given Lynn's knowledge of the ill treatment meted out to Jews, her views are shocking. She admitted to knowing about the 'horrors Jews suffer in Nazi lands. Stuffed into train & left till dead, packed in cells & steam turned on till dead etc.'[84] It is remarkable that in neutral Ireland with strict censorship Lynn knew about the Holocaust. Was it through her German friends? Perhaps knowledge about the final solution was more widespread than later commentators realise. Considering her regular complaints about the ill treatment of Irish political prisoners, it is paradoxical that she was not to the fore in articulating concerns about Jews. While she was concerned about sanitation, surely she did not wish to ethnically cleanse the Jews. Yet, it is clear from her diary entry of 1944 that she knew that there were Jews being murdered on the Continent. Lynn was not always compassionate even in the face of such horrors.

When US troops were stationed in Northern Ireland, Lynn suggested they had 'too much money' and 'immorality' was 'rampant'.[85] Not surprisingly, she was very antagonistic towards Churchill. 'He seems like Dev., can brook no opinion but his own.'[86] She was also very pointed in her assessment of the Allies generally, as well as sympathetic towards the Germans. Eight 'MPs etc have gone to see German prison camps 1st hand & all the horrors, when one thinks of what they did to us & U.S. to the natives, one knows their insincerity. Poor Germany almost squeezed in betw. enemies & surely they are no worse than the Allies.'[87] With Hitler's death Lynn suggested he was 'great in many ways.'[88] Despite the horrors brought on Europe by Hitler's policies, Lynn blamed the war on rampant 'barbarism' and, predictably, the fact that God was 'forgotten'.[89] Her eulogies of the Soviet Union in the 1930s disappeared in the following decades.

SAVE THE GERMAN CHILDREN SOCIETY

Immediately after the war there were large numbers of refugees, including children. Gradually, the horrors of the German regime were revealed. Lynn's friend and fellow paediatrician, Dr Bob

Collis, tended to the ill in the Belsen Concentration Camp and exposed the tragedy of the conditions there. Lynn thought his account of the camp was 'truly horrible, one can't believe that orderly people like the Germans could have tolerated such appaling conditions'.[90] Lynn redeemed herself by helping the Save the German Children Society which brought German refugees to Ireland after the war. The secretary of the Society, Isolde Farrell, sent a circular to Lynn about helping Germany as she wanted Lynn's help.[91] By mid October 1945, Lynn could delight in the fact that her St Ultan's colleague, Dr Kathleen Murphy, had 'launched her scheme for bringing over German children & placing them with families, with great eclat'.[92] The project was known as 'Operation Shamrock'.[93] Lynn became vice-president of the Society in 1948.[94] Collis's knowledge of the grim situation in central Europe was an advantage and he spoke to the Society about the conditions there.[95] Lynn's busy day was extended by Society meetings and she was put in charge of the north Dublin branch of the Society. With obvious delight, she noted that the efforts of the Society had 'aroused gt. enthusiasm'.[96] By September 1945 she reported that Áine Ceannt, the widow of the executed 1916 leader, Éamonn Ceannt, was 'at Killybegs seeing German children'.[97] Lynn knew Áine Ceannt through her work on behalf of the Irish White Cross which helped Irish children who were affected by the War of Independence and the Civil War.[98]

Inevitably, there were concerns about the religious make-up of the children, so much so that Roman Catholics were preferred. Lynn was critical of this attitude. 'The Friends [Society of Friends, the Quakers] have taken all the poor little Lutherans that the Irish Church failed to take, what a reflection!'[99] Eventually, in 1951, a German–Irish Society was established which Lynn helped to found.[100] However, while she wished to focus on welfare, the Society was 'all out for lectures, concerts, excursions & so on. No much thought of helping poor German displaced persons.'[101] Nonetheless, the Society surely helped to improve Irish–German relations in the 1950s.

NATIONAL BCG CENTRE

While the suffering associated with the Second World War was gradually made public, the tragedy of death from TB remained quiet, even shameful. Given the disease's association with poverty, it was usually hidden from view. Much of the credit for eliminating tuberculosis in Ireland has gone to the pioneering Minister for Health, Dr Browne. However, his political style tended to alienate people. Lynn thought he was 'really unfair to Med. profession & blames us for high death rate & because all have not v. best attention & really we have always done all possible for poor in hospitals etc. & only in govt. controlled places were they neglected. Dr Abrahamson [Professor of Medicine at the Royal College of Surgeons][102] said truly we weren't responsible for housing, feeding, resting the people.'[103] Browne's immensely popular autobiography, *Against the Tide*, failed to explain the views of the medical profession. Dr Malachy Powell saw the young physician as 'inexperienced, arrogant and fanatical'. Furthermore, Browne sneered that it 'was a measure of the resourcefulness of our opponents that they were able to mobilise a wealthy Jewish specialist named Abrahamson and a Protestant paediatrician named Colles [sic] in support of the bishops' opposition to the mother and infant service.' When Browne became Minister for Health, he managed, in one fell swoop, to attack many members of the medical profession while guest speaker at the Royal College of Surgeons of Ireland Biological Society inaugural meeting. 'Abrahamson and Collis, present in the audience, defended the profession with equal vehemence.'[104]

Nonetheless, Browne's social conscience and dynamism injected much-needed energy into the campaign to eliminate TB. Lynn thought highly of her St Ultan's colleague Dorothy Price, as she was 'kind' and 'sensible'.[105] It was Price who pioneered the introduction into Ireland of the BCG vaccine (Bacillus Calmette and Guerin) named after the two French scientists who discovered it. Having achieved success in St Ultan's, Price eventually convinced the medical profession of its effectiveness. BCG was introduced more widely in Ireland in the late 1940s. Price was not afraid to insist on her mode of vaccination for the elimination of TB. As she proudly announced to Dr Wallgren, who had pioneered BCG in Sweden, 'I had the Minister here twice & finally persuaded him to do what I wanted.'[106] Given that a large children's hospital was still badly needed, preventing disease was one way of trying to improve infant mortality rates. Price suggested to Dr Pearl Dunlevy, who administered the BCG at the Rotunda, that the need for children's hospital beds was 'being pressed home' in 1948.[107] Price and Lynn visited Browne in May 1949 in order to discuss the 'possibility of extending facilities for BCG vaccination throughout the country'.[108] Lynn was delighted when the BCG centre was opened at St Ultan's in June 1949; it was 'a day to be proud of'.[109] But Browne's impatience affected the St Ultan's centre. On a visit to Browne at his department, Lynn complained that he 'launched on us, that he thinks it time to make B.C.G. a national thing, paid for by rates and taxes, it would be an enormous task . . . Better go slow, but that's not Dr Browne.'[110] A few days later, the hospital received a letter from Browne, 'denying he was ever dictatorish in his speech, but everyone who heard him said he was Hitler again. He is so nice it is sad he can't brook opposition.'[111] Fundamentally the St Ultan's staff, particularly Lynn, wanted to choose their own colleagues.[112] After Price became ill, Dr John Cowell became the new director of the national BCG centre. He was 'like a son' to Lynn, so clearly he suited her.[113] The loss of control over appointments would have irked Lynn, and she is surprisingly critical of certain St Ultan's staff in her diaries. By 1950, when there were ninety cots at St Ultan's, Lynn could not exert the same control she had enjoyed in the 1920s.[114]

MOTHER AND CHILD

Browne was no stranger to friction. His ill-fated, if well-intentioned, attempts to provide medical care for all mothers and their children floundered in the midst of the medical profession's and the Catholic Church's opposition to what they saw as socialist medicine in the form of a Mother and Child Scheme. This scheme would have extended free medical care to mothers and their children.[115] Lynn was peeved when Dr Reddin, the Medical Officer of the Maternity and Child Welfare Scheme of the City of Dublin, announced that the new scheme was 'ready for action'. We, she pointed out, who 'started Baby treatment' were 'passed over'.[116] As in political life, when new plans were being enacted, those who had contributed to earlier pioneering activities were quickly forgotten. When Browne published the correspondence relating to the negotiations between the various parties, it exposed some politicians and churchmen. While many historians have heard the ecclesiastical chorus, they have also realised that the bishops were using the IMA's hymn sheet. Dermot Keogh observed that 'many years later the then Bishop of Ferns, Donal Herlihy, told me: "we allowed ourselves to be used by the doctors, but it won't happen again."'[117] Catholic ethics had been the rock on which an enlarged St Ultan's had perished in the 1930s. Likewise, the hierarchy's objections in the 1950s are an echo of the complaints voiced in the 1930s. The hierarchy claimed that the scheme could include advice on birth control, 'on which the Catholic Church had definite teaching.'[118] There were medical practitioners who would not be comfortable with the state-salaried physicians giving advice on child care and maternal health. Even more fundamentally, these physicians did not want to lose the fees from middle-class patients. 'The bishops' address to the government was not a protest against the mother-and-child scheme; it was an articulation of the private practitioners' case.'[119] Lynn was wary of Sean MacBride, Browne's colleague in government, and the son of Maud Gonne MacBride. He did not emerge with much credit from the controversy. 'I am not surprised for he is Madam's child', Lynn tellingly commented.[120] Yet for all the print expended on the Mother and Child Scheme, the late 1940s did initiate a greater awareness of the state's role in the improvement of public health. Lynn and her St Ultan's colleagues were part of that development.

Ironically the partial failure of the Mother and Child Scheme is seen as a triumph for the Catholic hierarchy. In fact, it was the medical profession with its desire to retain its middle-class patients which drove the opposition to the Scheme. Working-class patients, who were forced to use the dispensary system, had no choice of doctor, but their needs were not considered. While Lee has suggested that priests were 'strong farmers in cassocks',[121] their ecclesiastical superiors, the bishops, were the higher professions in episcopal garb. McQuaid's brother was a doctor and sometime president of the IMA. The class issues at stake in the Mother and Child Scheme have been overlooked in favour of a present-centred and somewhat simplistic Church versus State conflict. Most ironically of all, John Cooney's desire to paint McQuaid as all-powerful and panoptic has elevated the former archbishop. McQuaid failed to prevent a means tested Mother and Child Scheme being introduced by an adept Fianna Fáil government in 1953. He also failed to have all TB sanatoria under Catholic control. He may have lost medical battles, but he won the Catholic Children's Hospital crusade. 'His Grace's' hospital was opened in 1956 with the Catholic Archbishop of Dublin as the manager. Lynn's hopes for a multi-denominational hospital were never realised.

DEATH: 'I WAS BUSY BUT MY WORK IS SO SMALL.'

Despite being in her seventies, Lynn continued to do a lot of her travelling on her bicycle in the 1940s and '50s.[122] She also maintained contact with her nephew and nieces in Australia and mentioned receiving 'such a nice letter fr. Winsome', her niece, John Lynn's daughter.[123] Later she mentioned receiving 'lovely photos of the children' from Winsome.[124] Lynn's brother John returned to Ireland in the spring of 1948 and stayed with her until his death in March 1954. Despite the demands made by an elderly brother, Lynn was 'thankful' that she was 'able to mind him to the last'.[125] Clearly, she was the one he turned to as he rarely visited his sister Muriel in Warrenpoint. Indeed, by 1950, a rift had developed between Lynn and Muriel. She reported that Muriel did not want to see her brother and sister and was 'quite content to be separated from us all. In fact she seems to revel in it. Well, she doesn't know how it hurts.'[126] Characteristically, when Muriel became ill some months later, Lynn rushed to Warrenpoint to tend to her sister.[127] However, by Christmas all had been healed, since, as usual, Lynn went to Warrenpoint for the holiday. The contrast between Lynn and Muriel could not have been greater. While Lynn was a persistent republican, Muriel was wary of the Irish Republic. In many ways, Muriel's experiences were replicated by many Protestants who left the new Irish state after independence.

As a Protestant in a state that was overwhelmingly Catholic, Lynn provides insights into the views of a member of the minority. She noted that the anti-partition speakers were instructed to 'show how careful the 26 counties are of non R.Cs partly true & not altogether for in many things we would not get a look in'.[128] Yet Lynn shared the moral views of the majority. She thought a sermon that dealt with 'family life & how divorce has ruined it was excellent'.[129] Lynn's experience of medical politics in the 1930s, '40s and '50s, would have convinced her of the difficulties facing Protestants. She had seen how the Meath Hospital Board was overturned by the Knights of St Columbanus, who voted Catholics onto the Board.[130] She asked, 'Is it "Catholic Action"? Alas, alas.'[131] The Meath, like many hospitals under Protestant management, selected its staff from the supply of Trinity graduates. Catholic doctors therefore felt discriminated against. Lynn represented, as she wrote herself, 'Protestants who want to be Irish not west Britons . . . if we only could get at the people who filled S[t.] Mary's for the Wolfe Tone Service' in 1948.[132] It was Lynn's belief that patriotic Protestants had a role to play in the new Ireland.

Because of the restrictions of her gender, and, to a lesser extent, her denominational affiliation, Lynn was to become more of a witness than a participant in the emerging state. How much she could have done if she was a member of the Dáil is impossible to calculate. Perhaps she was able to do more outside the confines of parliamentary politics. As Finola Kennedy has noted, there were several Protestant women who were 'key figures in improving social conditions in twentieth-century Ireland'.[133] Like Lynn, Hilda Tweedy was particularly interested in the provision of school meals. As founder of the Irish Housewives' Association (IHA) she promoted the welfare of women and children. Yet, as with St Ultan's, the IHA was perceived as Protestant and therefore suspect. Lynn even suggested that there was 'a great need in the city of Dublin for a school for prospective fathers and mothers'.[134] As usual, the losers were those who needed nutrition.

Towards the end of her life, Lynn admitted, 'I was busy but my work is so small'. This may sum up her life, since so much of what she did were immeasurable small deeds, but for those she came in contact with, it made a big difference. Even a week before her 77th birthday, she admitted being busy with patients from ten in the morning until ten at night.[135] While in a pessimistic mood, she thought the world pursued 'godless futility'; yet the following day she happily noted that the Save the German Children Society was 'very alive . . . Things grow & do well.'[136] Lynn's very busyness kept her alive for so long. Her old friends, the Byrnes and the Nugents in County Wicklow, as well as her medical mentor, Moorhead, sustained her. Furthermore, republican friends like Síghle Humphreys provided her with that much-remembered link to her earlier political activities. Of course, some of the idealism of her earlier years had dissipated. Mary Kettle, a long-time friend and political soulmate, gave a 'great dissertation on all the benefits wh. have come since women got votes. It is true, but for my part I had thought it would have transformed the world & it didn't. I thought the same w[ou]ld. be when the British were gone, but that was a greater disappointment.'[137] Clearly, the political frustrations of living in the Irish Republic were greater than those that accompanied the partial attainment of gender equality. As Peter Hart has perceptively suggested, 'Revolutionary republicanism is probably the most female-dependent major movement in modern Irish history.'[138] Yet the work of these republican women is muted in histories of Ireland. Furthermore, the vital work performed by Lynn and other members of the Church of Ireland was not given full recognition in the new state. She was triply discriminated against as a female, Protestant, republican. However, unlike many others, Lynn enjoyed the comforts of a professional lifestyle.

Lynn was asked by an *Irish Times* journalist in 1951 what republican women did after 1916. She thought her 'motif' would be St Ultan's.[139] Just months before Lynn's death, Dr Virginia Apgar of Columbia University Medical School, who had published an article on evaluating newborn infants just two years previously, visited St Ultan's. Lynn suggested she was 'very pleasing & seemed interested'.[140] Apgar had graduated in 1933 and initially concentrated on anaesthesiology, becoming the first female full professor at Columbia University. Later she became interested in maternal and child health, hence her visit to St Ultan's. She invented the Apgar score which measured infant respiration and was crucial in the evaluation of infant needs.[141] Clearly, the impact of Lynn's work spread far beyond Ireland. Yet Lynn remained an Irish nationalist to the end. Her penultimate diary entry records her attendance at a commemoration ceremony for 1916. Appropriately, it was a 'beautiful day like 1916 was'. Later she prepared to visit her beloved Glenmalure.[142] Pearse suggested that he wanted to 'have a place in the heart of a child'.[143] While he is associated with educational progress, it is Lynn who was associated with caring for children.

Lynn was blessed that her maid Brigid was there at all times in the final years of her life. She died on 14 September 1955 at St Mary's Home in Ballsbridge, a home managed by the Church of Ireland. Lynn had been admitted to the home just a few months earlier and had written her will there. Not surprisingly, she left most of her money to her relations in Australia.[144] Furthermore, as a devoted republican she remained loyal to Wolfe Tone, the 'father' of 'Ireland's first republican movement'.[145] Lynn's will stipulated that her picture of Revd Matthew Young, Tone's tutor at Trinity,[146] and later Bishop of Clonfert in the midlands, should be donated to the National Museum. Lynn was buried in the family plot at Deansgrange in Dublin with full military honours. Her old nemesis de Valera attended. To the end, she remained committed to the ideals of the 1916 Rising, particularly its promise to cherish all the children of the nation.

Anne Jellicoe, one of the founders of Alexandra College, Lynn's Alma Mater, died in 1880. An anonymous obituarist romantically concluded that 'the night does not close on Mrs Jellicoe's life until the influence of her life passes from amongst us.'[147] Members of religious minorities were quietly significant in the history of Ireland and Lynn reflected Jellicoe's social commitment and vision. The writer Thomas Carlyle suggested in 1850 that 'before "dying" for your country, think, my friends, in how many quiet strenuous ways you might beneficially live for it.'[148] Lynn lived for Ireland. However, her quiet, strenuous work was quickly forgotten.[149]

NOTES

1 Noël Browne, *Against the Tide* (Dublin, 1986); James Deeny, *To Cure and To Care: Memoirs of a Chief Medical Officer* (Dublin, 1989).
2 The memoirs of Deeny make clear that he vehemently disagreed with Browne. John Horgan, *Noël Browne: Passionate Outsider* (Dublin, 2000). This important biography has one brief reference to St Ultan's and no reference to Dr Dorothy Stopford Price.
3 'James Deeny, 1906–1994', in John Quinn (ed.), *My Education* (Dublin, 1997), pp. 75–83, p. 79. Many influential Jesuits, such as Edward Cahill and Edward Coyne, provided the intellectual foundations of Catholic social teaching. The conclusion of the Deeny piece is revealing: 'I have a wonderful wife, who has given me a postgraduate course in humility. I am not very good at it yet. In fact, she says it's not working . . .'
4 Jones, *History of Tuberculosis*, p. 194.
5 Ibid., pp. 159–85.
6 Ibid., pp. 200 and 202.
7 Kennedy, *Cottage to Creche*, p. 197; see Cooney, *John Charles McQuaid*, for McQuaid's Ulster background.
8 John Duffy to John Charles McQuaid, 8 Nov. 1942, in McQuaid Papers, Government Box 4, AB8/B, DDA.
9 Greta Jones, 'review of T.M Healy, *From Sanatorium to Hospital: A Social and Medical Account of Peamount, 1912–1997'*, in *Irish Economic and Social History*, 2002, pp. 178–79, p. 179.
10 J.M. O'Donovan's career can be traced in the *Medical Directory*; O'Donovan to Price, 22 Feb. 1944, in Price Papers, 7537/9, TCD MS Dept.
11 O'Donovan to Price, 10 August 1944, Price Papers, 7537/37, TCD MS Dept.
12 Evelyn Bolster, *Knights of Columbanus* (Dublin, 1974), p. 84.
13 Ibid., p. 94.
14 Annick O'Brien, 'John Charles McQuaid and the fight against tuberculosis in the 1940s', BA dissertation, TCD, 2002, courtesy of the author.
15 Her book on childhood TB was reviewed favourably in the United States, and she received requests for advice and information from Australia, the United States and Britain. See Price Papers MS 7537, TCD MS Dept.
16 LD, 7 May 1940.
17 LD, 15 Oct. 1941.
18 LD, 28 Jan. 1944.
19 LD, 6 March 1942.
20 LD, 26 May 1943.
21 Gerard Fee, 'The effects of the Second World War on Dublin's low-income families, 1939–1945' (Ph.D., UCD, 1996), p. 153.
22 An unpublished study of Cork City during the Second World War suggests that 45 per cent of households were living below the poverty line; Enda Delaney, *Irish Emigration since 1921* (Dundalk, 2002) p. 25.

23 Till Geiger, 'Why Ireland needed the Marshall Plan but did not want it: Ireland, the sterling area and the European Recovery Program, 1847-8', in *Irish Studies in International Affairs*, vol. ii, 2000, pp. 193–215, p. 199.
24 Charles Clancy Gore, M.D., 'Nutritional standards of some working class families in Dublin, 1943', in *Journal of the Statistical and Social Inquiry Society of Ireland*, vol. 17, 1943–44, pp. 240–53, p. 253; Margaret Mitchell, 'The effects of unemployment on the social condition of women and children in the 1930s', in *History Workshop Journal*, Issue 19, (spring 1985), p. 111.
25 Frank McCourt, *Angela's Ashes: A Memoir of a Childhood* (London, 1996). Ferriter asserts that the 'begrudgers who insist Frank McCourt exaggerated the poverty of Limerick would find ample evidence of the stark poverty he described if they consulted Limerick Corporation's Medical Officer's reports from the era.' Diarmaid Ferriter, 'Suffer Little Children? The historical validity of memoirs of Irish childhood', in Joseph Dunne and James Kelly (eds), *Childhood and its Discontents: The First Seamus Heaney Lectures* (Dublin, 2002), pp. 69–105, p. 103. A trawl through the files of the local government board in the early 1920s suggests a world of diphtheria and dead donkeys. The latter were occasionally responsible for causing the former by infecting the water supply.
26 Anon., 'Some aspects of an improved medical service', in *The Journal of the Medical Association of Éire*, vol. 13, (Aug. 1943), p. 20, cited in Earner-Byrne, 'In respect of Motherhood', p. 52.
27 LD 17 Dec. 1943; James Deeny and Eric T. Murdock, 'Infant mortality in the city of Belfast', in *Journal of the Statistical and Social Inquiry Society of Ireland*, vol. 17, 1943–44, pp. 221–40.
28 LD, 26 and 27 May 1944.
29 LD, 6 June 1944.
30 LD, 12 Feb. 1945.
31 Mary Raftery and Eoin O'Sullivan, *Suffer the Little Children: The Inside Story of Ireland's Industrial Schools* (Dublin, 1999), p. 79.
32 LD, 20 March 1945.
33 James Kavanagh, 'Social activist', in *Studies*, vol. 87, no. 348, winter 1998, pp. 372–77, pp. 372–73.
This issue of *Studies* is devoted primarily to John Charles McQuaid.
34 Lindsey Earner-Byrne, '"In respect of motherhood": maternity policy and provision in Dublin City, 1922–56", Ph.D. thesis reports, *The History Review*, xiii (2002), pp. 194–98, p. 195.
35 Finola Kennedy, *Family, Economy and Government in Ireland*, Economic and Social Research Institute General Research Series, paper no. 143 (Dublin, 1989), p. 34.
36 LD, 28 Jan. 1945.
37 LD, 4 Feb. 1945.
38 Dónal Caird, 'A view of the revival of the Irish language', in *Éire-Ireland*, summer 1990, pp. 96–108.
39 Interview with Dr Dónal Caird, June 2000.

40 LD, 30 August 1940.
41 Jonathan Hamill, 'Childcare arrangements within the Belfast linen community, 1890–1930', in Whelan (ed.), *Women and Paid Work in Ireland, 1500–1930*, pp. 120–32, p. 131.
42 St Ultan's Annual General Meeting Minutes, 28 June 1942, SUA.
43 LD, 28 Oct. 1940.
44 LD, 15 Oct. 1942.
45 LD, 14 April 1948.
46 LD, 21 Jan. 1941.
47 LD, 20 Feb. 1941.
48 LD, 8 March 1943.
49 LD, 9 Nov. 1943.
50 LD, 11 March 1943. The devastation wrought by the fire is graphically illustrated in Diarmaid Ferriter, *'Lovers of Liberty'? Local Government in 20th century Ireland* (Dublin, 2001), p. 147. See also Mavis Arnold and Heather Laskey, *Children of the Poor Clares: The Story of an Irish Orphanage* (Belfast, 1985), for the perspectives of the orphans.
51 LD, 19 Oct. 1944; Susannah Riordain, '"A Political Blackthorn': Sean MacEntee, the Dignan Plan and the principle of ministerial responsibility', in *Irish Economic and Social History*, vol. 27, 2000, pp. 44–62.
52 LD, 14 March 1945.
53 Adrian Kelly, 'Catholic action and the development of the Irish welfare state in the 1930s and 1940s', in *Archivium Hibernicum*, liii, 1999, pp. 107–17.
54 LD, 22 Jan. 1941.
55 LD, 27 March 1942; for Price's career see Margaret Ó hÓgartaigh, 'Dr Dorothy Price and the elimination of childhood tuberculosis', in Joost Augusteijn (ed.), *Ireland in the 1930s: New Perspectives* (Dublin, 1999), pp. 67–82.
56 LD, 10 August 1942.
57 LD, 13 May 1942.
58 LD, 18 Dec. 1942.
59 LD, 22 March 1945.
60 St Ultan's General Board, 17 May 1945, in SUA
61 LD, 21 Feb. 1947.
62 LD, 28 Feb. 1947.
63 LD, 11 April 1940.
64 LD, 26 April 1940.
65 LD, 9 Sept. 1941.
66 LD, 5 Jan. 1942.
67 LD, 16 May 1945.
68 LD, 22 June 1945.
69 LD, 25 April 1947.
70 Dáil Éireann vol. 105, 1449–1450, 24 April 1947, the Sinn Féin Funds Bill; for a summary of the complications surrounding the finances of Sinn Féin, see Laffan, *The Resurrection of Ireland*, p. 450.

71 LD, 11 June 1949.
72 LD, 14 Nov. 1948.
73 LD, 16 Nov. 1948.
74 LD, 21 Nov. 1948.
75 LD, 1 Nov. 1951.
76 LD, 11 June 1940.
77 LD, 19 June 1941.
78 LD, 7 Nov. 1945.
79 LD, 26 Jan. 1942.
80 LD, 27 April 1942.
81 LD, 1 Oct. 1942.
82 LD, 16 March 1943.
83 LD, 12 May 1943.
84 LD, 16 April 1944.
85 LD, 20 August 1942.
86 LD, 5 Dec. 1942.
87 LD, 21 April 1945.
88 LD, 2 May 1945.
89 LD, 30 April 1945.
90 LD, 13 June 1945.
91 LD, 6 October 1945; Cathy Molohan, *Germany and Ireland, 1945–1955: Two Nations' Friendship* (Dublin, 1999), pp. 45–64.
92 LD, 17 Oct. 1945.
93 Dermot Keogh, *Jews in Twentieth-Century Ireland: Refugees, Anti-Semitism and the Holocaust* (Cork, 1998), pp. 209–12.
94 LD, 4 Nov. 1948.
95 LD, 20 Nov. 1945.
96 LD, 29 Nov. 1945.
97 LD, 3 Sept. 1946.
98 Lynn was a council member of the White Cross. Áine Ceannt, *The Story of the Irish White Cross* (Dublin, 1947), p. 9.
99 LD, 16 Sept. 1948.
100 Molohan, *Germany and Ireland*, pp. 79–82.
101 LD, 7 Feb. 1952.
102 Leonard Abrahamson's highly successful career is described in J.B. Lyons, *A Pride of Professors: The Professors of Medicine at the Royal College of Surgeons* (Dublin, 1999), pp. 255–65.
103 LD, 8 Nov. 1948.
104 Quoted in Lyons, *A Pride of Professors*, p. 264. 'Colles' was Bob Collis, a highly regarded paediatrician who was renowned for his work on behalf of the Dublin poor. Collis was a friend of Lynn who was also in favour of a large children's hospital. As discussed in chapter 3, their plans were scuppered by ecclesiastical and professional politics.
105 LD, 4 Sept. 1946.

106 Liam Price (ed.), *Dr Dorothy Price: An Account of Twenty Years' Fight against Tuberculosis in Ireland* (Oxford, 1957) p. 144.
107 Price to Pearl Dunlevy, 2 Sept. 1949, Dunlevy papers, courtesy of Mairead Dunlevy.
108 St Ultan's General Board Minutes, 19 May 1949, SUA.
109 LD, 20 June 1949.
110 LD, 13 Nov. 1950.
111 LD, 16 Nov. 1950.
112 'We don't want Drs on Staff that we didn't choose ourselves.' LD, 7 May 1951.
113 LD, 1 Feb. 1954.
114 St Ultan's General Board Minutes, 25 May 1950, SUA.
115 For a discussion of the Mother and Child scheme, see Ruth Barrington, *Health, Medicine and Politics in Ireland, 1900–1970* (Dublin, 1987), pp. 201–21. The role of the Irish Medical Association (IMA), originally the Medical Association of Éire, is brilliantly analysed in Eamonn McKee, 'Church-state relations and the development of Irish health policy: the mother-and-child scheme, 1944–53', in *Irish Historical Studies*, xxv, no. 98, Nov. 1986, pp. 159–94.
116 LD, 9 May 1950.
117 Keogh, *Twentieth-Century Ireland* p. 213.
118 J.H. Whyte, *Church and State in Modern Ireland, 1923–1970* (Dublin, 2nd edn, 1980), p. 214.
119 McKee, 'Church-state relations', p. 187.
120 LD, 12 April 1951.
121 Lee, *Ireland, 1912–1985*, p. 159.
122 'Did a lot on cycle.' LD, 3 Oct. 1946, when she was 72.
123 LD, 16 Oct. 1946. I am grateful to Lenore McKay, John Lynn's granddaughter, and the daughter of Winsome Lynn, for providing me with copies of Lynn's letters. Winsome Lynn was born in 1915.
124 LD, 17 Nov. 1952.
125 LD, 4 March 1954.
126 LD, 5 March 1950.
127 LD, 31 May 1950.
128 LD, 9 Feb. 1949.
129 LD, 23 March 1951.
130 Dr Stafford Johnson of the Knights of Columbanus, had sought an 'investigation' into the Meath Hospital: Peter Gatenby, *Dublin's Meath Hospital, 1753–1996* (Dublin, 1996), p. 122.
131 LD, 9–12 April 1949.
132 LD, 30 Nov. 1951.
133 Kennedy, *From Cottage to Crèche*, p. 263; Hilda Tweedy, *A Link in the Chain: The Story of the Housewives Association* (Dublin, 1992).
134 St Ultan's Annual General Meeting Minutes, 25 May 1950, SUA.
135 LD, 20 Jan. 1951.
136 LD, 13 and 14 August 1947.

137 LD, 15 March 1951.
138 Peter Hart, 'Definition: defining the Irish revolution', in Joost Augusteijn (ed.), *The Irish Revolution, 1913–1923* (Basingstoke and New York, 2002), pp. 17–33, p. 22. Richard English's essay, 'Socialism: socialist intellectuals and the Irish revolution' in the same volume does not even consider the role of women socialist intellectuals, many of whom, particularly Lynn, were far more pragmatic than their male republican counterparts.
139 LD, 5 and 15 June 1951; the article appeared in 'The Irish Woman's Diary', in the *Irish Times*, 15 June 1951.
140 LD, 14 April 1955; MacFarquhar Desmond, *Newborn Medicine and Society*, p. 266.
141 Ellen More, *Restoring the Balance: Women Physicians and the Profession of Medicine, 1850–1995* (Cambridge, Mass. and London, 1999), p. 180.
142 LD, 24 April 1955.
143 Cited in ffrench-Mullen obituary in St Ultan's Annual Report 1945, p. 12.
144 Will of Kathleen Lynn, 1/2/56, NAI.
145 Elliott, *Wolfe Tone*, p. 419.
146 Will of Kathleen Lynn, 1/2/56, NAI; Young 'was a gifted scholar, with Catholic tastes, and under such a polymath Tone's education would have been wider than suggested by the narrowness of the syllabus and examination system.' Elliott, *Wolfe Tone*, p. 19. It may be possible that Lynn heard about Bishop Young through Church of Ireland circles. The National Museum has no record of the donation of the Young picture, but they admitted that they did not keep catalogues in the 1950s.
147 Anon., 'The late Mrs Jellicoe', *Journal of the Women's Education Union*, 8 (1880), cited in Maria Luddy, *Women in Ireland, 1800–1918* (Cork, 1995), pp. 137–38, p. 138.
148 Thomas Carlyle (1850) quoted in Kevin Whelan, *The Tree of Liberty: Radicalism, Catholicism and the Construction of Irish Identity, 1760–1830* (Cork, 1996), p. 131.
149 In 1964 Sidney Gifford Czira (John Brennan) wrote about Lynn and ffrench-Mullen since the surgical unit was opened in St Ultan's in honour of Lynn in that year. She was described as a 'quiet, shy' woman who had shown 'remarkable courage and resolution'. The daughter of 'a Mayo vicar of strong Unionist principles' borrowed books on 'Irish history, literature and economics' from Helena Molony. 'From this schooling, Dr Lynn emerged a convinced Irish Republican and, as her character was a blend of practicality and idealism, she proved a most valuable recruit.' *Irish Independent*, 12 Nov. 1964; cited in Alan Hayes (ed), *The Years Flew By: Recollections of Madame Sidney Gifford Czira* (Galway, 2000), pp. 114–16.

CHAPTER SIX

Radical witness

> Love is patient, love is kind. It does not envy, it does not boast, it is not proud. It is not rude, it is not self-seeking, it is not easily angered, it keeps no record of wrongs. Love does not delight in evil but rejoices with the truth. It always protects, always trusts, always perseveres.
>
> St Paul's Letter to the Corinthians. The First Epistle of Paul to the Corinthians, chapter 13, versus 4–8

IT MAY SEEM STRANGE to begin an assessment of a radical feminist with a quotation from St Paul. He is hardly a feminist icon! However, theologians suggest that Paul was a firm believer in diversity and social action. Lynn, a reader of St Paul, shared his multi-cultural and multi-lingual outlook. Not surprisingly, she did not subscribe to his sexism. How does one assess such a varied and multi-cultured, as well as inflexible and divisive figure? Many of Lynn's activities were hidden yet she witnessed so much. Through her diaries one senses her desire to document the many activities and events she either witnessed or participated in.

What does Lynn represent? For some she was a radical, republican feminist, others take delight in her professional achievements. The Medical Registration Council Headquarters is known as Lynn House. Appropriately, it is in Rathmines, very close to the old site of St Ultan's and her home on Belgrave Road. Lynn was full of contradictions, a radical feminist who apparently did not approve of trousers. Fellow republican Máire Comerford thought that Lynn was 'quite an old-fashioned person' who 'persuaded Constance Markievicz to wear a skirt over her breeches in 1916'.[1] Her colleague Dorothy Price thought Lynn was 'a very charming lady of an old-fashioned type'.[2] Perhaps Lynn was a mixture of modernity and tradition.

Writing in the first half of the twentieth century, in her essay on medieval ideas about women, Eileen Power, a contemporary of Lynn, noted that the 'position of women is often considered as a test by which the civilisation of a country or age may be judged'. Furthermore, she pointed out that the 'position of women is one thing in theory, another in legal position, yet another in everyday life. In the Middle Ages, as now, the various manifestations of women's position reacted on one another but did not exactly coincide; the true position of women was a blend of all the three.'[3]

What was the position of Lynn and her contemporaries? Certainly, her life was a lot easier than those whose children she tended. For most women, a professional career was not an option.[4] Lynn had a disposable income, she could afford to attend concerts and plays. Her holidays were spent in Wicklow or Down, in Britain or on the Continent. This was a life that would have appealed to many. However, most could not afford it.

One of Lynn's contemporaries suggested that her 'biographer will find her name and very little more'.[5] Nothing could be further from the truth, as she left a large documentary legacy. In her diaries, she cheerfully, and occasionally venomously, comments on political enemies, 'Union Jacky' relations and awkward colleagues. Despite this large personal record, is it possible to judge the career and contribution of someone as diverse and multi-faceted as Dr Kathleen Lynn? This last chapter will analyse the entirety of her life, from Mayo beginnings to her death in Dublin. Was she unique, or one of the more active members of a generation of women who have been either eulogised or ignored? Trinity academic W. B. Stanford suggested that Protestants in the Irish Free State should 'lie low and say nothing'; this was not Lynn's philosophy.[6] The views of contemporaries and her own comments are suggestive of a life which was full of faith, hope, charity and frustration. Remarkably, Lynn was an icon for some even during her own life. She noted comically in 1934 that an 'old woman in Albert Place has me on her wall next to Willie Cosgrave!!! Did one ever hear the like.'[7]

Lynn was born in 1874 and died in 1955. Ireland changed dramatically during her life. Just three years before Lynn was born, there were 339,000 Episcopalians and 3,616,000 Roman Catholics in Ireland.[8] In 1946, there were 2,786,000 Roman Catholics and 125,000 Episcopalians in the Irish Free State. Lynn was, however, part of a slowly increasing number of professional women. When she was born there were no female physicians. By 1951, there were 499 women in the Irish Republic enumerated as medical practitioners. Women's share of the medical profession in the 1950s, when they constituted more than 15 per cent of doctors, compares favourably with international figures. In 1950, women still only made up 6 per cent of the profession in the United States.[9] During Lynn's lifetime women moved increasingly into professional careers, they gained the vote and some became prominent in national life. Yet, for many, the attainment of political independence was a disappointment. Dónal Caird suggested that 'Cumann Gaelach na hEaglaise was the institution in which many found the vehicle to express their loyalties to Protestantism and to an independent republican state and to the Irish language.'[10]

Lynn was more 'Linn Féin' than Sinn Féin.[11] She was a 'self help' person, who sought action in the face of inertia. People take what they want from her. She saw, and commented on, the Mé Féin (myself) philosophy in independent Ireland. Perhaps she expected too much of an impoverished new state. Yet most of her long life was spent as a citizen of the United Kingdom, since she was 48 by the time the Irish Free State was established. While she sought international links, particularly with Continental Europe and the United States, the new state remained very dependent economically on Britain. Like most republicans, her disdain for Britain was both consistent and irrational.

REPUBLICANISM

Republicanism was traditionally seen as a 'manly calling'. Yet the civic virtue espoused by male republican thinkers was clearly enacted by women. Martha McTier, sister of William Drennan, one of the founders of the United Irishmen, personified the 'sense of industry as well as social responsibility' which republicans tried to inculcate. 'Her republicanism, based on the notion that true civic virtue required public service, compelled her to engage in one of the few public activities left to a middle-class woman in the nineteenth century – philanthropy.'[12] So it is with Lynn, whose work in medicine was politicised philanthropy.

The United Irishmen sought to include those who endured discriminatory legislation. However, the United Irishmen patently ignored the female half of the population. Fraternity, as usual, triumphed over liberty and equality. The United Irishmen had eighteenth-century attitudes. It would be unrealistic to expect them to be concerned with twentieth-century issues. The late eighteenth-century focus on citizenship may be compared with the late nineteenth- and early twentieth-century debates about women as citizens. Lynn's involvement in the Irish Citizen Army can be seen as her attempt to ensure that women were part of the political world. Both the 1790s and the 1910s were concerned with political equality and independence. There was also a strong millenarian sense in both eras. The belief that the world could be changed through revolution was an ethos shared by many of the protagonists in the United Irishmen and Sinn Féin. Lynn shared these optimistic visions of a brave new republican world. Yet women were excluded from many republican activities. As Luddy has noted, 'while the 1790s were a time when the rights of Irish men were constantly being urged there was little concern with the rights of women.'[13]

It has been suggested that, as well as 'liberty, fraternity, and equality, the French revolutionaries declared for motherhood'.[14] In the immediate aftermath of the late eighteenth century and early twentieth century revolutions, there was a particular emphasis on motherhood. This was particularly evident in Germany and Italy in the 1930s. The great loss of life in the 1790s and 1910s was one source of this ideology. Though she was no fascist, Lynn shared the fascist's cult of motherhood, but she was aware of the difficulties inherent in raising large families with small incomes. At any rate, Lynn knew that the demands of the motherhood movement placed particular stress, both economic and medical, on women. Unlike many, she had a pragmatic response. Her work in St Ultan's was an indication of her commitment to mother and infant health, as well as a welcome professional boost for female physicians.

Lynn's generation of women was very aware of their exclusion from many aspects of Irish life. They too alerted the public, through the pages of *The Irish Citizen*, to the inequalities endured by women. However, female discrimination persisted for many years. In 1923, Lynn wrote: 'Fr Caffrey of Francis St read paper re Women's work. Was he asleep 25 yrs?'[15] Lynn remained committed to her feminist socialist ideals in the new state. However, both Sinn Féin and the United Irishmen were conservative revolutionaries.

SOCIALISM

James Connolly provided Lynn with many of her socialist ideas. Over twenty years after his death she was reading his 'Socialism Nationalist & Religion' and proclaiming it to be 'wonderful'.[16] However, Lynn was very much a product of her class and she was aware of this. 'Strange how those who are working will spend 12/6 [twelve shillings and six pence, or sixty-two and a half pence] on Sunday excursion while so many starve & still we often do same ourselves', she wrote.[17] Despite her obvious concern for others, she did not deprive herself of entertainment. Yet her medical activities surely helped many. Her concern was always for the poor. It 'is really terrible when the unemployed are driven like starving rats fr. pillar to post & nothing is done for them. Couldn't all who have 3 meals give one for those who have none,' she pleaded.[18]

For her patients, Lynn was their salvation. Her diaries are suffused with concerns for her patients and friends. She was, at various times, and sometimes simultaneously, a political radical, pioneering paediatrician, cultured traveller, energetic philanthropist and uncompromising ideologue. Before attempting an assessment of her life, we might ask how Lynn assessed her own life. She places the same date annually in her diary, so that she may comment on her activities a year ago on that date. She is often wistful, occasionally disappointed and frequently determined to reassure herself. Nonetheless, throughout her diaries she constantly admonishes herself. The puritanical element in her make-up ensured that she demanded a lot of herself both physically and intellectually. Many nationalists were influenced by religious ideology. Lynn could be dismissive of non-Christians: 'Terrible tales of Japanese, wholesale bombing of Chinese towns, slaying multitudes of civil population. Well what can one expect those who know not God will do anything.'[19] At the St Ultan's Annual General Meeting in 1954, the writer John D. Sheridan echoed the views of Lynn by suggesting that 'our real assets were spiritual, love, prayer, devotion and confidence'.[20]

At the end of her life Lynn was not living in the secular, socialist, republican state she sought. Professionally, she was a highly-regarded general practitioner, though seen as somewhat eccentric with her fresh air fetish. However, politically and economically she was disappointed with the Irish Republic. Lynn survived these various disappointments through a deep sense of spirituality.

SPIRITUALITY

One of the major motivations in Lynn's life was her deep spirituality. She was a pantheist who drew particular comfort from nature. Her relationship with God and the saints was consoling and fortifying. During the War of Independence, after attending a religious service at Doulough, she wrote: 'I never realised more fully the communion of saints, our own Irish saints were very much present in that spot, sacred for so long & our prayers were one for our country's freedom.'[21] She was also a devout, if critical, member of the Church of Ireland. Though she had many Roman Catholic friends and was ecumenical in her outlook, she did not share the theology of Catholicism. On one occasion, she complained that a service was 'too Romish in parts.'[22] However, Dr Dónal Caird thought that her beliefs were quite High Church, so she would have been close to Catholicism in some respects. It is not surprising that she was devoted to St Brigid, the female patron saint who transcended Reformation divisions. On 1 February 1926, the saint's day, she wrote: 'Oh! The joy of the Gaelic & the feeling of the nearness of S. Brigid.'[23] Eight years later she consoled herself with the thought that 'we know S. Brigid & those beyond work for

Éire's good'.[24] Brigid's work in tending to the sick and establishing an independent community of women is a mirror of Lynn's work.[25]

We may describe Lynn's spiritual outlook as close to the Céile Dé (companions of God), an eighth-century Church reform movement, which placed an emphasis on simplicity, companionship and frugality. They emphasised an individual relationship with God. Clearly Lynn was a regular converser with God. Her diaries are filled with DGs (Deo Gratias, thanks be to God). This profound spirituality provided her with the strength and endurance to persist, despite difficulties. It was also a justification, however partisan, for her political perspective.

Lynn was far from charitable towards political enemies. Like her spiritual ancestors, she was 'an ascetic, severe on herself'.[26] The puritanical element amongst revolutionaries has been observed by others, and is very evident in Lynn's diaries. Garvin suggests that 'asceticism is a common characteristic of the modern revolutionary leader'.[27] However, this tendency also ensured that Lynn could be severe towards others (though some of her assessments are possibly accurate). Count Plunkett, an early leader of Sinn Féin, was 'a crank'.[28] Dan Breen's book on his republican activities was 'disguising'.[29] Peadar O'Donnell, a fellow socialist, was 'the great humbug'.[30]

Historians have described republicans, like Lynn, of the 1920s, as 'advanced nationalists'. Lynn saw the pro-Treatyites as, in a sense, remedial nationalists. Those who opposed the Treaty did not fare much better. For Lynn, the anti-Treatyites who eventually entered the Dáil as Fianna Fáil in 1927 were remedial republicans.[31] She had no time for the strategic republicanism of Fianna Fáil. Empty formulas meant nothing to her. Lynn's refusal to compromise made her a poor politician. Intellectual and ideological gymnastics were not her forte. Hence, she failed politically, but was a trusted and loyal friend. Given the multitude of problems facing Ireland after the Second World War, socialism was unable to thrive. As Lee has noted, 'sectarianism in Belfast and nationalism elsewhere suffocated socialism culturally as well as ideologically'.[32]

Lynn's clear sympathy for militarism should not be discounted. However, the 1910s were deeply militaristic, with the First World War as well as the military events of the 1916–23 period in Ireland.

While, strictly speaking, she was not a combatant in 1916, she clearly sympathised with, and aided, the rebels. Her medical expertise was used to harass and humiliate the authorities in Ireland.

In the medical republic of St Ultan's the shared interest in paediatrics helped make health a public issue. However, there was little evidence of republican equality of treatment with nurses earning half the income of the administrator, and the portress worst paid of all.[33] While political citizenship was much sought after, economic citizenship was much more valuable. However, it was not easily attainable.

CONCLUSION

In 1956 de Valera agreed to open a youth hostel for An Óige in Glenmalure which was dedicated to Lynn.[34] This hostel had been Lynn's summer cottage. In his speech, he suggested that Lynn should be always remembered. He also pointed out that he had 'no intimate or personal knowledge of the social and charitable work in which he knew Dr Kathleen Lynn had engaged; but he had personal knowledge of the work she did for the independence of the country in the political sphere'. His impression was that 'she was one who worked very much more than she talked'. Furthermore, Lynn was 'one of those persons to whom if everything was not pure white it was black. But she was most charitable in her views of others.' (Clearly de Valera was not reading her diaries!) He went on to point out that she 'worked for the nation as a whole, and I hope people throughout the country will also remember her'. Yet it was de Valera's protective policies which ensured that the contribution of women like Lynn would be muted in the Irish Republic. Furthermore, the focus on political affairs has clouded the achievements of those who sought to improve people's daily lives. De Valera's women were supposed to dance at the cross roads not dissect in the operating room!

It would be very easy to paint a hagiographical picture of Lynn given her indefatigable work for others, as well as her charitable disposition. Lynn was 'Christlike' in her compassion and concern, but she could be demanding, inflexible and impatient. She was venomous but not vengeful. There is no doubting her capacity for loving others.

Lynn's work, with its successes and failures, suggests that she was devoted to the nation. Her philosophy may be traced back to her childhood and early development in Mayo. She lived during a patriot era, when, for some, patriotism was a fatal attraction. She was fortunate to survive the tempestuous 1910s and early 1920s. Moreover, Lynn was then able to enact her personal, medical philosophy in St Ultan's Hospital for Infants, which became a women's medical republic. She was not, in the phrase of Tom Paine, the eighteenth-century radical, a 'sunshine patriot'. On the contrary, her patriotism was of the practical variety. Máire Comerford described her as 'our most practical practising revolutionary'.[35] Lynn's philosophy was based on love of nation. Her work was designed to improve the lives of others. In a reference for her young colleague, Dr Rose Barry, who began working in the hospital in 1950, Lynn praised Barry's ability to 'make even the most downhearted infant smile'.[36] This quality was valued.

Lynn helped to change the face of paediatric medicine. However, she was not alone. Other prominent physicians such as Bob Collis, James Deeny and Dorothy Price also played their part in making children's health a national issue.[37] Her work was revolutionary in the context of a new state more concerned with political issues. Fittingly, it was through her work for others that she is remembered. In the words of Máire Comerford:

> Dr Lynn was a woman of action, and she had a full life, and there must have been a few days in that life when she did not combine in her own person the ideal set forth in the Proclamation of 1916 – 'Cherish all the children of the nation equally.' Children needed love, she held, so it was a rule of the hospital that every child was an individual, and must know himself, or herself, loved.[38]

Her colleague, Ursula Hurley, remembered visiting Lynn as she lay dying in St Mary's. Worried about St Ultan's, Hurley asked how they could survive without Lynn. Lynn's simple response was that 'everyone can be done without'. Hurley also noted that Lynn was 'always in command of herself and of other people'.[39] Lynn displayed her civic competence and commitment in a whole range of activities. She wanted others to continue her work. When Barbara Stokes began working at St Ultan's, Lynn thought that 'God arranged for us to have Dr Stokes on Board. She has all teaching requirements at her finger tips.'[40] Montessori teaching was initially designed for mentally disabled children. Stokes was to be awarded the Kennedy Prize for her work with disabled children many years after Lynn's death.

In May 1956, at the first St Ultan's Annual General Meeting after Lynn's death, Dr Rose O'Doherty delivered a eulogy on Lynn:

> Though indefinably reserved, she was never aloof, always approachable. She loved the garden. Above all else she loved the babies. Hail, rain or snow, she visited them every day, not only for her own patients but every baby in the hospital. She knew the importance of love and the sense of being wanted. This was instilled into the nurses.[41]

Lynn gave her diaries to her relative, William Wynne, in 1955. He was to imbibe her eccentricity and philanthropic commitment. In order to make a point at one sermon, he rode a bicycle up the aisle of the church. Wynne established the Samaritans in Ireland in 1959. The ancient Greeks believed that if you influenced someone, you were immortal. Lynn lives on.

NOTES

1 *Irish Press*, 6 November 1969, in Press Cuttings Scrapbook, SUA.
2 Price quoted in León Ó Broin, *Protestant Nationalists in Revolutionary Ireland: The Stopford Connection* (Dublin, 1985), p. 204.
3 Eileen Power, *Medieval Women* (Cambridge, 1995), p. 1.
4 The lives of ordinary women in the first forty years of the Irish Free State have been analysed by Caitriona Clear, in *Women of the House: Women's Household Work in Ireland, 1922–1961* (Dublin, 2000). See, in particular, chapter 5, which discusses aspects of pregnancy and childbirth.
5 *Irish Press*, 6 November 1969, in Press Cuttings Scrapbook, SUA.
6 Quoted in Alan Megahey, *The Irish Protestant Churches in the Twentieth Century* (London and New York, 2000), p. 116.
7 LD, 26 March 1934.

8 All the census statistics are taken from the Census of Ireland Reports.
9 More, *Restoring the Balance: Women Physicians and the Profession of Medicine, 1850–1995*, p. 186.
10 Quoted in James McLoone (ed.), *Being Protestant in Ireland: Papers presented at the 32nd Annual Summer School of the Social Study Conference at St Kieran's College, Kilkenny, 4–8 August 1984* (Naas, 1984) p. 60. For the career of Lil Nic Dhonnchadha, who was active in Cumann Gaelach, see Risteárd Ó Glaisne, *De bhunadh Protastúnach nó rian Chonradh na Gaeilge* (Dublin, 2000), pp. 291–343.
11 'Linn Féin' means by ourselves.
12 Nancy Curtin, 'Women and eighteenth-century Irish Republicanism', in Mary O'Dowd and Margaret MacCurtain (eds), *Women in Early Modern Ireland* (Edinburgh, 1991), pp. 137–39, p. 143. For the correspondence between William Drennan and Martha McTier, see Jean Agnew (ed.), *The Drennan-McTier Letters, 1776–1819*, 3 vols (Dublin, 1998–9).
13 Maria Luddy, 'The Women's History Project', in *Women's Studies Review: Oral History and Biography, Volume 7*, pp. 67–80, p. 70.
14 Michael West, 'Nationalism, race and gender: the politics of family planning in Zimbabwe, 1957–1990', in *Social History of Medicine*, vol. 7, no. 3, Dec. 1994, pp. 447–71, p. 447.
15 LD, 13 Oct. 1923.
16 LD, 2 March 1937.
17 LD, 20 May 1925.
18 LD, 30 Nov. 1927.
19 LD, 28 Sept. 1937.
20 St Ultan's Annual General Meeting minutes, 27 May 1954, SUA.
21 LD, 3 August 1919.
22 LD, 18 April 1924.
23 LD, 1 Feb. 1926.
24 LD, 1 Feb. 1934.
25 St Ultan was a kinsman of St Brigid, see Angela Bourke, 'Irish stories of weather, time and gender: Saint Brigid', in Marilyn Cohen and Nancy Curtin (eds), *Reclaiming Gender: Transgressive Identities in Modern Ireland* (New York, 1999), pp. 14–30.
26 *Irish Press* 6 November 1969, Press Cuttings Scrapbook, SUA.
27 Tom Garvin, *Nationalist Revolutionaries* (Oxford, 1987), p. 156.
28 LD, 14 Sept. 1923.
29 LD, 27 Feb. 1925.
30 LD, 14 Sept. 1925.
31 Her comments in the 1930s and '40s on Fianna Fáil are a clear indication of her disappointment with the anti-Treaty party.
32 J.J. Lee, 'Worker and society since 1945', in Dónal Nevin (ed.), *Trade Unions and Change in Irish Society* (Cork, 1980), pp. 11–25, p. 17.
33 For a discussion of the working conditions of nurses, see Ó h'Ógartaigh 'Flower Power and "Mental Grooviness": nurses and midwives in early twentieth century Ireland', pp. 133–47.

34 The following is based on de Valera's file on Lynn in the de Valera Papers, UCDA.
35 *Irish Press*, 6 November 1969, Press Cuttings Scrapbook, SUA.
36 Lynn reference for Dr Rose Barry, 12 July 1950, courtesy of Dr Rose Barry.
37 I have learned much from Dr Lindsey Earner-Byrne, who has written a Ph.D. thesis at UCD on motherhood in the Irish Free State, Dr Vanessa Rutherford who has written a Ph.D. thesis at the National University of Ireland, Maynooth, on childhood in late nineteenth- and twentieth-century Ireland, and Dr Frances Carruthers who has written a Ph.D. on Lady Aberdeen, also at NUI Maynooth. I am grateful for their generosity.
38 *Irish Press*, 11 Nov. 1969, Press Cuttings Scrapbook, SUA.
39 Interview with Ursula Hurley, July 2000.
40 LD, 3 March 1948.
41 St Ultan's Annual General Meeting, 31 May 1956, SUA.

Bibliography

PRIMARY SOURCES

MANUSCRIPT

Ireland
Adelaide and Meath Hospitals, incorporating the National Children's Hospital [Tallaght Hospital]
Adelaide Hospital Minutes

Allen Library, O'Connell Schools, Dublin
Madeleine ffrench-Mullen files
Kathleen Lynn files

Dublin City Archives, Dublin
Minutes of the Rathmines and Rathgar Urban District Council
Leahy, Bríd *Dublin City Archives: Abstract of political career of Dr Kathleen Lynn as a member of the Rathmines and Rathgar Urban District Council, 1920–1930* (Dublin, 2000)

Dublin Diocesan Archives
William Walsh Papers
Edward Byrne Papers
John Charles McQuaid Papers

Military Archives, Cathal Brugha Barracks, Dublin
Witness Statements: Alice Barry, Brian Cusack, Áine Ceannt, Richard Hayes, Kathleen Lynn, Helena Molony and Kathleen O'Brennan
Captured Documents Lot 120

National Archives of Ireland
1911 Census, Dublin 60/26
D/E [Department of Local Government] 2/475

Bibliography

Chief Secretary's Office Papers 13503/16
Department of An Taoiseach, S.3147, S1369–10, S5074B, S2547A
Will of Kathleen Lynn, 1/2/56

National Library of Ireland
Sinn Féin Standing Committee Minute Book (Jan 1918–May 1919) Photostat
Lynn, Kathleen 'Report on Influenza Epidemic, March 1919', in Sinn Féin Election Pamphlets
Hayes, Richard and Kathleen Lynn *Public Health Circulars, no. 1*, (Sinn Féin Public Health Department, Dublin, February, 1918)
Sinn Féin Re-Organisation Meeting in the Mansion House, 11 Feb. 1923.
Sinn Féin Re-Organising Committee, 4 July 1924
Sinn Féin Clár [Programme], Árd Fheis, 1926
Sinn Féin Election Poster
Sinn Féin Pamphlet, Árd Fheis, 8 April 1919

National Library of Ireland, Manuscripts Department
Hanna Sheehy Skeffington Papers
Minute Book of Cumann na dTeachtaire
Robert Barton Scrapbook
Áine Ceannt/Lily O'Brennan Papers
Rosamund Jacob Diary

Queen's University Belfast, Special Collections
Belfast Eugenics Society Minutes

Registry of Deeds, Dublin
Folio 2826, Co. Wicklow

Representative Church Body Library, Dublin
File on Robert Lynn, RCBL MS 61/2/15.

Royal College of Physicians in Ireland, Dublin
Kirkpatrick Biographical Archive
Lynn Diaries
St Ultan's Hospital Papers

Trinity College, Dublin, Manuscripts Dept
Dorothy Stopford Price Papers MS 7537

University College Dublin Archives
Royal College of Science Registers
Éamon de Valera Papers
Sighle Humphreys Papers
Kathleen O'Brennan Papers

England
National Archives, Kew, London
WO 364/2185/ Service file on John Lynn
CO 904/207/251, Kathleen Lynn file

USA
Burns Library, Boston College
Wilson Pamphlets

Rockefeller Archives, Sleepy Hollow, New York
Kathleen Lynn Correspondence

St John's Seminary Library, Boston
Boston Pilot

Schlesinger Library, Radcliffe Institute, Harvard
Martha Eliot Papers

PRINTED

Agnew, Jean (ed.) *The Drennan-McTier Letters, 1776–1819*, 3 vols (Dublin, 1998–99)
Anon. 'Some aspects of an improved medical service', *The Journal of the Medical Association of Éire*, vol. 13, (Aug. 1943)
Anon. 'The late Mrs Jellicoe', *Journal of the Women's Education Union*, 8 (1880).

Annual Reports of the Board of Superintendence of the Dublin Hospitals, with Appendices, 1920–21, 1921–22.
Cameron, Charles *Reminiscences of Sir Charles A. Cameron, C.B.* (Dublin and London, 1913).
Census of Ireland *Reports*, 1881, 1891, 1901, 1911, 1926, 1936, 1946, 1951 and 1956.
Childers, Erskine *Military Rule in Ireland: A series of Eight Articles contributed to the Daily News March – May, 1920* (Dublin, 1920)
Clancy Gore, Charles, M.D. 'Nutritional standards of some working class families in Dublin, 1943' *Journal of the Statistical and Social Inquiry Society of Ireland*, vol. 17, 1943–44, pp. 240–53.
Coey Bigger, Edward *The Carnegie United Kingdom Trust: Report on the Physical Welfare of Mothers and Children: vol. iv, Ireland, 1917* (Dublin, 1917).
Connolly, James *The Reconquest of Ireland* (Dublin, Irish Transport and General Workers Union, 1934, first published in 1915).
Dáil Debates (Dublin, 1922–56)
Day, Susanne *The Amazing Philanthropists* (London, 1916).
Deeny, James and Eric T. Murdock 'Infant mortality in the city of Belfast', *Journal of the Statistical and Social Inquiry Society of Ireland*, vol. 17, 1943–44, pp. 221–40.
Groag Bell, Susan and Karen Offen (eds) *Women, the Family and Freedom: The Debate in the Documents* (Stanford, 1983).
Hayes, Alan (ed) *The Years Flew By: Recollections of Madame Sidney Gifford Czira* (Galway, 2000)
Irish Women's Suffrage Federation Report for 1915
Jex-Blake, Sophia MD *Medical Women: A Thesis and A History* (second edition, Edinburgh and London, 1886).
Litton, Helen (ed) *Kathleen Clarke Revolutionary Woman. My Fight for Ireland's Freedom* (Dublin, 1991).
Ministry of Health, *Annual Report of the Chief Medical Officer*, 1919–1920, vol. xvii, 1920, Cmd.978.
National Children's Hospital [Harcourt Street] Annual Report 1928.
National University of Ireland Calendars, 1909–1955.
Reports of the Department of Local Government and Public Health
Reports of the Executive Committee of the Irish Women's Suffrage and Local Government Association for 1902–16

Reports of Registrar General
Robertson Commission 1902, Appendix to 3rd Report Parliamentary
    Paper, vol. xxxii, cd. 1229
Royal University of Ireland Calendars
The Medical Directory, 1876–1955.
WNHA Golden Jubilee, 1907–1957. The Women's National Health
    Association of Ireland (Dublin, 1957).

Newspapers

Bean na hÉireann
Cumann na mBan
Evening Herald
Evening Mail
Freeman's Journal
Honesty
Irish Citizen
Irish Independent
Irish Press
Irish Worker
Sinn Féin
The Irish Times
The Times
Weekly Irish Times

Periodicals

Alexandra College Magazine
British Medical Journal
Catholic Bulletin
Dublin Journal of Medical Science
Irish Ecclesiastical Record
Irish Journal of Medical Science
Irish Monthly
Irish Nursing News
Journal of the American Medical Association
Lancet
Medical Press
Medical Press and Circular

St Stephen's
The British Journal of Nursing

Material in private ownership
Madeleine ffrench-Mullen scrapbook
Angela Russell Scrapbook
Pearl Dunlevy Papers
Winsome Lynn Papers

SECONDARY SOURCES

Anderson, W.K. *James Connolly and the Irish Left* (Dublin, Portland and Melbourne, 1993).

Arnold, Mavis and Heather Laskey *Children of the Poor Clares: The Story of an Irish Orphanage* (Belfast, 1985).

Augusteijn, Joost (ed.) *Ireland in the 1930s: New Perspectives* (Dublin, 1999).

—— (ed.) *The Irish Revolution, 1913–1923* (Basingstoke and New York, 2002).

Barrington, Ruth *Health, Medicine and Politics in Ireland, 1900–1970* (Dublin, 1987).

Berg, Maxine 'Foreword: Eileen Power, 1889–1940', in Eileen Power, *Medieval Women* (Cambridge, 1995), pp. ix–xxvi.

Breathnach, Eibhlín 'A History of the Movement for Higher Education in Dublin, 1860–1912' (MA, UCD, 1981).

Blom, Ida 'Equality and the threat of war in Scandinavia, 1884–1905' in T.G. Fraser and Keith Jeffery (eds), *Men, Women and War* (Dublin, 1993), pp. 100–18.

Bock, Gisela 'Poverty and mothers' rights in the emerging welfare states', in Francoise Thébaud (ed.), *A History of Women in the West: Volume V Towards a Cultural Identity in the Twentieth Century* (Harvard, Cambridge and London, 1994), pp. 402–30.

Bolster, Evelyn *Knights of Columbanus* (Dublin, 1974).

Bourke, Angela 'Irish stories of weather, time and gender: Saint Brigid', in Marilyn Cohen and Nancy Curtin (eds), *Reclaiming Gender: Transgressive Identities in Modern Ireland* (New York, 1999), pp. 14–30.

Bourke, Angela, Siobhán Kilfeather, Maria Luddy, Margaret Mac Curtain, Gerardine Meaney, Máirín Ní Dhonnchadha, Mary O'Dowd and Clair Wills, (eds), *The Field Day Anthology of Irish Writing: vol. iv: Irish Women's Writing and Traditions* (Cork, 2002).

Boyle, Denis *A History of Meath County Council, 1899–1999: A Century of Democracy in Meath* (Navan, 1999).

Browne, Alan 'Antiquarian book browsing', Valedictory Lecture as President of the History Section of the Royal Academy of Medicine in Ireland, 4 December 2002.

Browne, Noël *Against the Tide* (Dublin, 1986).

Butler Kahle, Jane (ed.) *Women in Science: A Report from the Field* (Philadelphia, 1985)

Caird, Dónal 'A view of the revival of the Irish language', *Éire-Ireland*, summer 1990, pp. 96–108.

Carruthers, Frances 'The organisational work of Lady Ishbel Aberdeen, marchioness of Aberdeen and Temair (1857–1939)' (Ph.D., National University of Ireland, Maynooth, 2001).

Ceannt, Áine *The Story of the Irish White Cross* (Dublin, 1947).

Clark, Linda *Schooling the Daughters of Marianne* (New York, 1984).

Clear, Caitriona 'Review of Margaret Ward, *The Missing Sex: Putting Women into Irish History*', *Linen Hall Review* 1987, p. 81.

—— *Women of the House: Women's Household Work in Ireland, 1922–1961* (Dublin, 2000).

Coakley, Davis *Irish Masters of Medicine* (Dublin, 1992).

Coleman, Marie 'The origins of the Irish Hospitals' Sweepstake', *Irish Economic and Social History*, vol. xxix, 2002, pp. 40–56.

—— '"They also served": the Role of Cumann na mBan in the War of Independence – the Evidence from County Longford', in *PaGes. Postgraduate Research in Progress*, UCD Arts Faculty, Volume 5, 1998, pp. 31–42.

Collis, Robert *To be a Pilgrim* (London, 1975).

Cooney, John *John Charles McQuaid: Ruler of Catholic Ireland* (Dublin, 1999).

Crookes, Gearóid *Dublin's Eye and Ear: The Making of a Monument* (Dublin, 1993).

Cullen Owens, Rosemary *A Social History of Women in Ireland, 1870–1970* (Dublin, 2005).

―― *Smashing Times: A History of the Irish Women's Suffrage Movement, 1889–1922* (Dublin, 1984 and 1995).

Cullen, Mary (ed.) *1798: 200 Years of Resonance: Essays and Contributions on the History and Relevance of the United Irishmen and the 1798 Revolution* (Dublin, 1998).

―― (ed.), *Girls Don't Do Honours: Irish Women and Education in the Nineteenth and Twentieth Centuries* (Dublin, 1987).

―― 'Anna Maria Haslam (1829–1922)', in Mary Cullen and Maria Luddy (eds), *Women, Power and Consciousness in Nineteenth-Century Ireland: Eight Biographical Studies* (Dublin, 1995), pp. 161– 96.

Curtin, Nancy, 'Women and eighteenth-century Irish Republicanism', in Mary O'Dowd and Margaret MacCurtain (eds), *Women in Early Modern Ireland* (Edinburgh, 1991), pp. 137–39.

Daly, Mary E. (ed.) *County and Town: One Hundred Years of Local Government in Ireland* (Dublin, 2001).

―― '"An Atmosphere of Sturdy Independence": the State and the Dublin Hospitals in the 1930s' in Elizabeth Malcolm and Greta Jones (eds), *Medicine, Disease and the State* (Cork, 1999) pp. 234–52.

―― 'Local appointments', in Mary E. Daly, (ed.), *County and Town: One Hundred Years of Local Government in Ireland* (Dublin, 2001), pp. 45–55.

―― 'Women in the Irish Free State, 1922–39: the interaction between politics and ideology', in Joan Hoff and Maureen Coulter (eds), *Irish Women's Voices. Past and Present. Journal of Women's History* vol. 6, no. 4/vol. 7, no. 1 (winter/spring), (Indiana, 1995), pp. 99–116.

―― *Dublin, the Deposed Capital* (Cork, 1984).

―― *Industrial Development and Irish National Identity, 1922–39* (Dublin, 1992).

Day, Roddy, Fionnuala Waldron, Tommy Maher and Pauric Travers *Time Traveller 1* (Dublin, 1996).

Deeny, James *The End of an Epidemic: Essays in Irish Public Health, 1935–65* (Dublin, 1995).

―― *To Cure and To Care: Memoirs of a Chief Medical Officer* (Dublin, 1989).

Delaney, Enda *Irish Emigration since 1921* (Dundalk, 2002).

Dickson, David, Dáire Keogh and Kevin Whelan (eds) *The United Irishmen: Republicanism, Radicalism and Rebellion* (Dublin, 1993).

Donnelly, Brian and Margaret Ó hÓgartaigh, 'Medical Archives for the Socio-Economic Historian', in *Irish Economic and Social History*, 2000, vol. 27, pp. 66–72.

Dunlevy, Pearl 'Kathleen Lynn FRCSI, Patriot Doctor' in the *Irish Medical Times*, December 4, 1981.

Dunne, Joseph and James Kelly (eds) *Childhood and its Discontents: The First Seamus Heaney Lectures* (Dublin, 2002).

Dunwoody, Janet 'Child Welfare', in David Fitzpatrick (ed.), *Ireland and the First World War* (Dublin, 1986) pp. 69–75.

Earner-Byrne, Lindsey '"In Respect of Motherhood": an Irish Catholic Social Service, 1930–1954', paper presented to the Irish Historical Society, November 1999.

—— '"In respect of motherhood": maternity policy and provision in Dublin city, 1922–1956' (Ph.D., UCD, 2001).

—— '"In respect of motherhood': maternity policy and provision in Dublin City, 1922–56", Ph.D. thesis reports, *The History Review*, xiii (2002), pp. 194–98.

—— *Mother and Child: Maternity in Dublin, 1922–71* (Manchester, 2006).

Elliott, Marianne *Wolfe Tone: Prophet of Irish Independence* (New Haven and London, 1989).

Evans, David 'Tackling the "Hideous Scourge": the creation of venereal disease treatment centres in early twentieth-century Britain', *Social History of Medicine*, vol. 5, no. 3, December 1992, pp. 413–33.

Fahey, Tony, 'Housing and Local Government', in Mary E. Daly (ed.), *County and Town: One Hundred Years of Local Government in Ireland* (Dublin, 2001), pp. 120–29.

Fearon, William 'The national problem of nutrition', *Studies*, March 1938, vol. 27, pp. 15–24.

Fee, Gerard 'The effects of World War II on Dublin's low-income families, 1939–1945' (Ph.D., UCD, 1996).

Ferriter, Diarmaid, *The Transformation of Ireland, 1900–2000* (London, 2004).

—— 'Local government, public health and welfare in twentieth-century Ireland', in Mary E. Daly (ed.), *County and Town: One*

Hundred Years of Local Government in Ireland (Dublin, 2001), pp. 109–19.
—— 'Lovers of Liberty?' *Local Government in 20th century Ireland* (Dublin, 2001).
—— 'Suffer Little Children? The historical validity of memoirs of Irish childhood', in Joseph Dunne and James Kelly (eds), *Childhood and its Discontents: The First Seamus Heaney Lectures* (Dublin, 2002), pp. 69–105.
—— 'Review of Finola Kennedy, *Cottage to Creche: Family Change in Ireland*, *The Economic and Social Review*, vol. 33, no. 2, summer/autumn, 2002, pp. 259–62.
Finegan, John, (ed.), *Anne Devlin: Patriot and Heroine* (Dublin, 1992).
Finn, Irene, 'Women in the medical profession in Ireland, 1876–1919', in Bernadette Whelan (ed.), *Women and Paid Work in Ireland, 1500–1930* (Dublin, 2000), pp. 102–19.
Fitzpatrick, David (ed.) *Ireland and the First World War* (Dublin, 1986).
Fraser, T.G. and Keith Jeffery (eds), *Men, Women and War* (Dublin, 1993).
Froggatt, Peter 'Competing Philosophies: the "Preparatory" Medical Schools of the Royal Belfast Academical Institution and the Catholic University of Ireland, 1835–1909', in Greta Jones and Elizabeth Malcolm (eds), *Medicine, Disease and the State in Ireland, 1650–1940* (Cork, 1999), pp. 59–84.
Garvin, Tom *1922: The Birth of Irish Democracy* (Dublin, 1996).
—— *Nationalist Revolutionaries* (Oxford, 1987).
Gatenby, Peter *Dublin's Meath Hospital, 1753–1996* (Dublin, 1996).
Geiger, Till 'Why Ireland needed the Marshall Plan but did not want it: Ireland, the sterling area and the European Recovery Program, 1847–8', *Irish Studies in International Affairs*, vol. ii, 2000, pp. 193–215.
Hamill, Jonathan 'Childcare arrangements within the Belfast linen community, 1890–1930', in Bernadette Whelan (ed.), *Women and Paid Work in Ireland, 1500–1930* (Dublin, 2000) pp. 120–32.
Hart, Peter 'Definition: Defining the Irish revolution', in Joost Augusteijn (ed.), *The Irish Revolution, 1913–1923* (Basingstoke and New York, 2002) pp. 17–33.
Horgan, John *Noël Browne: Passionate Outsider* (Dublin, 2000).

Jackson, Alvin *Ireland, 1798–1998* (London, 1999).

—— 'J.C. Beckett: politics, faith, scholarship', *Irish Historical Studies*, vol. xxxiii, no. 130, Nov. 2002, pp. 129–50.

Jones, Greta *'Captain of all these men of death': The History of Tuberculosis in Nineteenth and Twentieth Century Ireland* (Amsterdam and New York, 2001).

—— 'Eugenics in Ireland: The Belfast Eugenics Society', *Irish Historical Studies*, vol. xxviii, no. 109, (May 1992), pp. 81–95.

—— 'Marie Stopes in Ireland – The Mothers' Clinic in Belfast, 1936–47', *Social History of Medicine*, vol. 5, no. 2, 1992, pp. 255–77.

—— 'The Rockefeller and medical education in Ireland in the 1920s', *Irish Historical Studies*, vol. xxx, no. 120, Nov. 1997, pp. 564–80.

—— 'Review of T.M. Healy, *From Sanatorium to Hospital: A Social and Medical Account of Peamount, 1912–1997*', *Irish Economic and Social History*, 2002, pp. 178–79.

Jordan, Donald *Land and Popular Politics in Ireland: County Mayo from the Plantation to the Land War* (Cambridge, 1994).

Kavanagh, James 'Social activist', *Studies*, vol. 87, no. 348, winter 1998, pp. 372–77.

Kelly, Adrian 'Catholic action and the development of the Irish welfare state in the 1930s and 1940s', *Archivium Hibernicum*, vol. liii, 1999, pp. 107–17.

Kennedy, Finola *Family, Economy and Government in Ireland*, Economic and Social Research Institute General Research Series, paper no. 143 (Dublin, 1989).

—— *Cottage to Crèche: Family Change in Ireland* (Dublin, 2001).

Keogh, Dermot *Twentieth-Century Ireland: Nation and State* (Dublin, 1994).

—— *Jews in Twentieth-Century Ireland: Refugees, Anti-Semitism and the Holocaust* (Cork, 1998).

—— *The Vatican, the Bishops and Irish Politics, 1919–39* (Cambridge, 1986).

Knirck, Jason '"Ghosts and Realities": female TDs and the Treaty debate', *Éire-Ireland*, winter 1997, vol. xxxii, no. 4, pp. 170–94.

Laffan, Michael *The Resurrection of Ireland: The Sinn Féin Party, 1916–1923* (Cambridge, 1999).

Lalor, Brian (ed.) *Encyclopaedia of Ireland* (Dublin, 2003).
Law, Cheryl *Suffrage and Power: The Women's Movement, 1918–1928* (London and New York, 1997).
Lee, J.J. 'Worker and society since 1945', in Dónal Nevin (ed.), *Trade Unions and Change in Irish Society* (Cork, 1980) pp. 11–25.
—— *Ireland, 1912–1985: Politics and Society* (Cambridge, 1989).
Lehane, Aidan C.S.Sp., 'The Visitor', *Studies*, winter, 1998, vol. 87, no. 348, pp. 392–95.
Levenson, Leah and J.H. Natterstad *Hanna Sheehy-Skeffington, Irish Feminist* (Syracuse, 1986).
Lewis, Jane *The Politics of Motherhood: Child and Maternal Welfare in England, 1900–1939* (London, 1980).
Luddy, Maria (ed.) *Women in Ireland, 1800–1918: A Documentary History* (Cork, 1995 and 1999).
—— 'The Women's History Project', *Women's Studies Review: Oral History and Biography, Volume 7*, pp. 67–80.
Lynch, Kathleen 'The universal and particular: gender, class and reproduction in second-level schools', in *UCD Women's Studies Forum Working Paper*, no. 3, 1987.
Lyons, J.B. *A Pride of Professors: The Professors of Medicine at the Royal College of Surgeons in Ireland, 1813–1985* (Dublin, 1999).
—— *Brief Lives of Irish Doctors* (Dublin, 1978).
MacCurtain, Margaret 'Women, The Vote and Revolution', in Margaret Mac Curtain and Donncha Ó Corráin (eds), *Women in Irish Society, the historical dimension* (Dublin, 1978), pp. 46–57.
MacCurtain, Margaret and Donncha Ó Corráin (eds) *Women in Irish Society: The Historical Dimension* (Dublin, 1978).
Macdona, Anne (ed.) *From Newman to New Woman: UCD Women Remember* (Dublin, 2001)
MacFarquhar Desmond, Murdina *Newborn Medicine and Society. European Background and American Practice (1750–1975)* (Austin, 1998).
Magill, Isabel 'A social history of T.B. in Belfast' (D.Phil., University of Ulster at Jordanstown, 1992).
Maguire, Maria 'The development of the Welfare State in Ireland in the postwar period' (Ph.D., European University Institute, 1985).
Mahon, Bríd *While the Grass Grows: Memoirs of a Folklorist* (Cork, 1998).

Malcolm, Elizabeth 'Anne Devlin: the heroine as laundress?', *History Ireland* winter, 1998, pp. 9–10.

Markell Morantz-Sanchez, Regina, *Sympathy and Science: Women Physicians in American Medicine* (Oxford, 1985).

McCoole, Sinéad *No Ordinary Women: Irish Female Activists in the Revolutionary Years, 1900–1923* (Dublin, 2004).

McCourt, Frank *Angela's Ashes: A Memoir of a Childhood* (London, 1996).

McDowell, R.B. and D.A. Webb, *Trinity College Dublin, 1592–1952: An Academic History* (Cambridge, 1982).

McDowell, R.B. *Crisis and Decline: Southern Unionists in Ireland* (Dublin, 2000).

McKee, Eamonn 'Church-state relations and the development of Irish health policy: the mother-and-child scheme, 1944–53', *Irish Historical Studies*, vol. xxv, no. 98, Nov. 1986, pp. 159–94.

McLoone, James (ed.) *Being Protestant in Ireland. Papers presented at the 32nd Annual Summer School of the Social Study Conference at St Kieran's College, Kilkenny 4–8 August 1984* (Naas, 1984).

McManus, Ruth *Dublin, 1910–1940: Shaping the City & Suburbs* (Dublin, 2002).

Medical Council *Newsletter*, June 1997.

Meenan, F.O.C. *Cecilia Street: The Catholic University School of Medicine, 1855–1931* (Dublin, 1987).

Megahey, Alan *The Irish Protestant Churches in the Twentieth Century* (London and New York, 2000).

Migdal Glazer, Penina and Miriam Slater *Unequal Colleagues: The Entrance of Women into the Professions, 1890–1940* (London, 1987).

Miller Solomon, Barbara, *In the Company of Educated Women. A History of Women and Higher Education in America* (New Haven, 1985).

Mitchell, David *A 'Peculiar' Place: The Adelaide Hospital, Dublin. Its Time, Places and Personalities, 1839–1989* (Dublin, 1989).

Mitchell, Margaret 'The effects of unemployment on the social condition of women and children in the 1930s', *History Workshop Journal*, 19, (spring 1985), pp. 109–20.

Mitchell, Susan L. *Red-Headed Rebel: Poet and Mystic of the Irish Cultural Renaissance* (Dublin, 1998).

Mohr, Peter D. 'Dr Catherine Chisholm (1879–1952) and the Manchester Babies' Hospital (Duchess of York)', *Transactions of the Lancashire and Cheshire Antiquarian Society*, vol. 94, 1998, pp. 95–110.

Mokyr, Joel 'Why "More Work for Mother?": Knowledge and household behaviour, 1870–1945', *The Journal of Economic History*, March 2000, vol. 60, no. 1, pp. 1–41.

Molohan, Cathy *Germany and Ireland, 1945–1955: Two Nations' Friendship* (Dublin, 1999).

Morash, Christopher *A History of Irish Theatre, 1601–2000* (Cambridge, 2002).

More, S. Ellen *Restoring the Balance: Women Physicians and the Profession of Medicine, 1850–1995* (Cambridge, Mass. and London, 1999).

Morgan, Austen *James Connolly: A Political Biography* (Manchester, 1988).

Morrissey, Thomas J. *Towards a National University: William Delany SJ (1835–1924). An Era of Initiative in Irish Education* (Dublin, 1983).

Nevin, Dónal (ed.) *Trade Unions and Change in Irish Society* (Cork, 1980).

Novick, Ben *Conceiving Revolution: Irish Nationalist Propaganda during the First World War* (Dublin, 2001).

Ó Broin, León *Protestant Nationalists in Revolutionary Ireland: The Stopford Connection* (Dublin, 1985).

Ó Dochartaigh, Tomás *Cathal Brugha: A Shaol is a Thréithe* (Dublin, 1969).

Ó Glaisne, Risteárd *De bhunadh Protastúnach nó rian Chonradh na Gaeilge* (Dublin, 2000) pp. 291–343.

Ó hÓgartaigh, Margaret '"Is there any need of you?" Women in medicine in Ireland and Australia', in Special Issue of *Australian Journal of Irish Studies, vol. 4, Remembered Nations, Imagined Republics: Proceedings of the Twelfth Irish-Australian Conference, Galway, June 2002*, Louis de Paor, Maureen O'Connor and Bob Reece (eds) 2004, pp. 162–171.

—— 'Archival sources for the history of professional women', *Irish Archives*, vol 6, 1999, pp. 23–5.

—— 'Dr Dorothy Price and the elimination of childhood tuberculosis', in Joost Augusteijn (ed.), *Ireland in the 1930s: New Perspectives* (Dublin, 1999), pp. 67–82.

—— 'Emerging from the educational cloisters: educational influences on the development of professional women', *PaGes. Postgraduate Research in Progress*, vol. 3, 1996, pp. 113–23.

—— 'Flower Power and "Mental Grooviness": nurses and midwives in early twentieth-century Ireland', in Bernadette Whelan (ed.), *Women and Paid Work in Ireland, 1500–1930* (Dublin, 2000), pp. 133–47.

—— 'Mother Columba Gibbons of the Loreto Convent in Navan and author of the ballad "Who fears to speak of Easter Week"', *Ríocht na Midhe: Records of the Meath Archaeological and Historical Society*, vol. xvi, 2005, pp. 189–193.

—— 'St Ultan and Ardbraccan', *Ríocht na Midhe: Records of the Meath Archaeological and Historical Society*, vol. xiv, 2003, pp. 230–41.

—— 'St Ultan's, A Women's Hospital for Infants', *History Ireland*, summer 2005, pp. 36–9.

—— 'The Babies' Clubs in Ireland and the Children's Bureau in the US', in Chester Burns, Ynez Violé O'Neill, Philippe Albou and José Gabriel Rigau-Pérez (eds) *Proceedings of the 37th International Congress on the History of Medicine* (University of Texas Medical Branch, Galveston, Texas, 2001), pp. 99–103.

—— 'Women in Medicine, 1877–2000', in Brian Lalor (ed.) *Encyclopaedia of Ireland* (Dublin, 2003), p. 1148.

—— 'Women in University Education in Ireland: The Historical Background', in Anne Macdona (ed.), *From Newman to New Woman: UCD Women Remember* (Dublin, 2001), pp. 3–11.

—— *Dr Kathleen Lynn and Maternal Medicine* (Rathmines, Ranelagh and Rathgar Historical Association, Dublin, 2000).

—— 'A medical apppointment in County Meath', *Ríocht na Midhe: Records of the Meath Archaeological and Historical Society*, vol. xvii, 2006, pp. 266–70.

Ó Maitiú, Séamus *Rathmines Township, 1847–1930* (Dublin, 1997).

—— *Dublin's Suburban Towns* (Dublin, 2003).

O'Brien, Annick 'John Charles McQuaid and the Fight against Tuberculosis in the 1940s', BA dissertation, TCD, 2002.

O'Connor, Anne and Susan M. Parkes *Gladly Learn and Gladly Teach: A History of Alexandra College and School, Dublin 1866–1966* (Dublin, 1983).

O'Donnell, Frank Hugh *The Ruin of Education in Ireland* (London, 1902).

O'Dowd, Mary and Margaret MacCurtain (eds) *Women in Early Modern Ireland* (Edinburgh, 1991).

O'Neill, Marie *From Parnell to De Valera: A Biography of Jennie Wyse Power 1858–1941* (Dublin, 1991).

—— *Grace Gifford Plunkett and Irish Freedom: Tragic Bride of 1916* (Dublin, 2000).

O'Neill, T. P., 'From famine to near famine', *Studia Hibernica*, vol. 1, 1961, pp. 161–71.

Pašeta, Senia *Before the Revolution: Nationalism, Social Change and Ireland's Catholic Elite, 1879–1922* (Cork, 1999).

Perrin Behringer, Marjorie 'Women's role and status in the sciences: an historical perspective', in Jane Butler Kahle (ed.), *Women in Science: A Report from the Field* (Philadelphia, 1985), pp. 4–26.

Power, Eileen *Medieval Women* (Cambridge, 1995).

Preston, Margaret H. *Charitable Words: Women and the Language of Charity in Nineteenth-Century Dublin* (Westport, Connecticut, 2004).

Price, Liam (ed.) *Dr Dorothy Price: An Account of Twenty Years' Fight against Tuberculosis in Ireland* (Oxford, 1957).

Quinn, John (ed.) *My Education* (Dublin, 1997).

Raftery, Judith 'Professional advice-giving and infant welfare', *Journal of Australian Studies*, June, 1995, pp. 66–78.

Raftery, Mary and Eoin O'Sullivan *Suffer the Little Children: The Inside Story of Ireland's Industrial Schools* (Dublin, 1999).

Regan, Nell 'Helena Molony (1883–1967)', in Mary Cullen and Maria Luddy (eds), *Female Activists: Women and Change, 1900–1960*, pp. 141–68.

Riordan, Susannah '"A Political Blackthorn": Sean MacEntee, the Dignan Plan and the principle of ministerial responsibility', *Irish Economic and Social History*, vol. 27, 2000, pp. 44–62.

Roberts, Shirley *Sophia Jex-Blake: A Woman Pioneer in Nineteenth-Century Medical Reform* (London, New York, 1993).

Ruane, Medb 'Kathleen Lynn (1874–1955)', in Mary Cullen and Maria Luddy (eds), *Female Activists: Irish Women and Change, 1900–1960* (Dublin, 2001), pp. 61–88.

Rutherford, Vanessa 'Childhood in late nineteenth and twentieth-century Ireland' (Ph.D., National University of Ireland, Maynooth, 2002).

Ryan, Louise (ed.) *Irish Feminism and the Vote. An Anthology of the Irish Citizen Newspaper, 1912–1920* (Dublin, 1996).

—— '"Furies"' and "Die-hards"': Women and Irish Republicanism in the Early Twentieth Century', *Gender and History*, vol. 11, no. 2, July 1999, pp. 256–75.

Sheehy Skeffington, Andrée *Skeff: The Life of Owen Sheehy Skeffington, 1909–1970* (Dublin, 1991).

Statistical Yearbook of Ireland 2001 (Dublin, 2001).

Taillon, Ruth *When History was Made: The Women of 1916* (Belfast, 1996).

Te Brake, Janet 'Irish peasant women in revolt: the Land League years', *Irish Historical Studies*, May 1992, vol. xxvii, no. 109, pp. 63–80.

Thébaud, Francoise (ed.) *A History of Women in the West: Volume V, Towards a Cultural Identity in the Twentieth Century* (Harvard, Cambridge and London, 1994).

Travers, Pauric *Eamon de Valera* (Dublin, 1994).

Tweedy, Hilda *A Link in the Chain: The Story of the Irish Housewives Association 1942–1992* (Dublin, 1992).

Valiulis, Maryann Gialanella 'Toward "The Moral and Material Improvement of the Working Classes": The Founding of the Alexandra College Guild Tenement Company, Dublin, 1898', *Journal of Urban History*, vol. 23, no. 3, March 1997, pp. 295–314.

Walsh, Oonagh *Anglican Women in Dublin. Philanthropy, Politics and Education in the Early Twentieth Century* (Dublin, 2005).

Ward, Margaret 'The League of Women Delegates & Sinn Féin', *History Ireland*, autumn 1996, pp. 37–41.

—— *Unmanageable Revolutionaries: Women and Irish Nationalism* (Dublin, 1989).

Webster, Charles 'Healthy or Hungry Thirties', *History Workshop*, 13, spring 1982, pp. 110–29.

West, Michael 'Nationalism, race and gender: the politics of family planning in Zimbabwe, 1957–1990', *Social History of Medicine*, vol. 7, no. 3, Dec. 1994, pp. 447–71.

Whelan, Bernadette (ed.) *Women and Paid Work in Ireland, 1500–1930* (Dublin, 2000).

Whelan, Kevin 'The Politics of Memory', in Mary Cullen (ed.), *1798: 200 Years of Resonance: Essays and Contributions on the History and Relevance of the United Irishmen and the 1798 Revolution* (Dublin, 1998), pp. 143–60.

—— *The Tree of Liberty: Radicalism, Catholicism and the Construction of Irish Identity, 1760–1830* (Cork, 1996).

White, Jack *Minority Report: The Protestant Community in the Irish Republic* (Dublin, 1975).

Whyte J.H. *Church and State in Modern Ireland, 1923–1970* (Dublin, second edition, 1980).

Wilson, Adrian 'Conflict, consensus and charity: politics and the provincial voluntary hospitals in the eighteenth century', *English Historical Review*, June 1996, pp. 599–619.

INTERVIEWS
Rose Barry
Alan Browne
Dónal Caird
Brigid Dirrane
Pearl Dunlevy
Ursula Hurley
William Wynne

Index

Abbey Theatre, 20, 77, 112
Aberdeen, Ishbel Maria Gordon, Lady, 66, 70
Abrahamson, Leonard, 133, 143
Abt, I.A., 88
Adelaide Hospital, 5, 11–13, 71
Albert Edward, Prince of Wales, 8
Alexandra College, 9–12, 15, 66, 70–1, 139
American Red Cross, 48
Anderson, W.K., 20
Andrews, Marion, 67, 70
Anglo-Irish Treaty, 46–8, 85, 152
An Óige, 80, 92, 153
Apgar, Virginia, 138–9
Arbour Hill, 41
Ardbraccan, 69, 74, 112
Ardilaun, Sir Arthur Guinness, Lord, 7–8
Ashe, Thomas, 22, 34
Association for Women's Rights, 65

Babies' Clubs, 66, 70, 80, 82
Bacillus Calmette and Guerin: see BCG vaccine
Baker, Josephine, 82
Baldoyle, 75
Ballsbridge, 139
Ballymahon, 7
Ballyroan, 122
Barry, Alice, 22, 67, 70, 72, 79, 87, 98–101, 105
Barry, Eileen, 49
Barry, Kevin, 49
Barry, Rose, 154
BCG vaccine, 133–4
Bean na hÉireann, 3, 5
Belfast, 67, 72, 76, 79, 101, 120
Belfast Eugenics Society, 70
Belgium, 3, 112
Bell, Elizabeth, 126
Belsen, 132, 143
Berg, Maxine, 14
Beveridge Plan, 121–2, 124
Bigger, Edward Coey, 75–6
Birmingham, Ambrose, 11–12
birth control: see contraception
Black and Tans, 83
Blackrock College, 97, 103
Bodenstown, 2, 33
Bodkin, Thomas, 74

Bolster, Evelyn, 122
Boston (Massachusetts), 82
Brangan, Eileen, 93
breastfeeding, 75, 80–1
Breen, Dan, 152
Brennan, John, 145
Brigid, St, 87, 151–2, 156
Browne, Alan, 115
Browne, Noël, 119–20, 122, 133–5, 139
Brugha, Caitlín, 43, 61
Brugha, Cathal, 34, 46, 58, 61
Byrne family, 138
Byrne, Archbishop Edward, 93, 96–104, 121

Cahill, Edward, 139
Caird, Dónal, 3, 83, 90, 125–6, 148, 151
Cameron, Charles, 41
Canada, 81
Caribbean, 75
Carlyle, Thomas, 139
Carroll, Maeve, 3
Carson, Sir Edward, 75
Carson, Lady (Ruby), 75
Cat and Mouse Act (1913), 22
Catholic Action, 120, 137
Catholic Church: and refugee children, 132; power in Irish Free State of, 92–4, 114; and medical services, 97–8, 120–2, 127–8, 134–7; and St Ultan's Hospital, 73, 86, 96, 99–104; and social services, 125; social teaching of, 140
Catholics and Catholicism, 11, 12, 22, 148, 151
Catholic Social Service Conference, 120, 125
Catholic University Medical School: see under University College, Dublin
Cavan, 127
Ceannt, Áine, 35, 48, 52, 77, 83, 132
Ceannt, Éamonn, 132
Cecilia Street Medical School: see under University College, Dublin
Céile Dé, 152
Celtic Cross Association of Chicago, 77, 78

charitable activities, 6, 7, 21, 33, 64, 92
Chicago, 77
Child Health Council, 125
children and child care, 1–3, 51–3, 56, 63–7, 69, 73, 78, 92, 108, 113, 121, 154–5; Irish White Cross and, 48; in Limerick, 141; among refugees, 131–2; tuberculosis among, 128
Children's Act, 73
children's allowances, 106–7, 127
Children's Bureau (US), 82
China, 151
Chisholm, Catherine, 43, 76–7
Christian Brothers Archive, 4
Churchill, Winston, 47, 129, 131
Church of England, 93
Church of Ireland, 1, 3, 8, 71, 73–4, 116, 126, 138–9, 145, 148, 151
City Hall, 18, 24, 25, 26
Clancy Gore, Charles, 124
Clark, Linda, 9
Clarke, Harry, 74
Clarke, Kathleen, 27, 28, 33, 35, 48
Clarke, Tom, 27, 116
Clear, Caitriona, 46
Clemenceau, Georges, 45
Clongowes College, 119–20
Coiste na dTeachtaire, 35, 37
Coláiste Móibhí, 126
Colbert, Cornelius, 29
Collins, Michael, 34, 47
Collis, Robert, 94, 98, 131–3, 143, 154
Coltsford, 32
Columbia University, 139
Comerford, Máire, 146, 154
Communism, 107, 121, 130
Conditions of Employment Act 1936, 108
Cong, 6–8, 32, 36, 83
Connolly, James, 1–2, 18, 21, 23–5, 33, 38, 46, 51, 56, 150
Connolly, Seán, 24, 25, 26, 83
conscription, 39–40
Constitution of Ireland (1937), 92, 93, 110–11
Contagious Diseases Acts, 39

Index

contraception, 93, 101–3, 135
Cooke, Frances Margaret, 14
Cooney, John, 136
Corcoran, Timothy, 106
Cork, 67, 85, 121, 139
Cosgrave, Mary, 123
Cosgrave, W.T., 47, 84–5, 109, 147
county councils, 59
Cowell, John, 134
Coyne, Edward, 139
Craig, Sir James, 47
Crumlin, 104, 105, 127
Cuffe, Bridget, 14
Cumann Gaelach na hEaglaise, 57, 90, 125–6, 148, 156
Cumann na dTeachtaire, 34–5, 38–40, 55, 59, 69
Cumann na mBan, 18, 20, 24, 28, 43, 56
Cumann na nGaedheal, 47, 50, 51, 110, 111
Cusack, Brian, 32
Custom House, 119
Czira, Sidney Gifford, 145

Dáil Éireann, 44, 46, 50, 52, 92, 97, 108, 129–30, 137, 152
Daly family, 33
Daly, Mary E., 97, 104
Daly, P.T., 73
Davitt, Michael, 7
Day, Susanne, 85, 91
Deansgrange, 139
Deeny, James, 119–20, 124, 139, 154
Defence of the Realm Regulations, 41
Delaney, William, 10
Derry, 79
Despard, Charlotte, 62
De Valera, Éamon, 34, 46, 57–8, 74, 110–11, 129–31, 139, 153
Dickson, Winifred, 12
diphtheria, 141
divorce, 137
domestic science, 66
Dougan, Nan, 72, 126
Down, County, 147
Dowth, 69
Drennan, William, 148
Drumcliffe, 6
Dublin, 1, 5, 67–8, 72, 76, 95, 135; housing in, 85; mortality rates in, 15, 54; poverty and the poor in, 15, 21, 84, 98, 103, 119, 123, 126, 143
Dublin, County, 66
Dublin Castle, 18, 25–8, 30, 41
Dublin Civic Museum, 63
Dublin Corporation, 54, 67, 80, 108
Dublin Lockout (1913), 20, 21
Dublin Watch Committee, 38
Duffy, John, 120, 121

Dunbar-Harrison, Letitia, 93
Dundee, 68
Dundrum, 3
Dunlevy, Pearl, 94, 134
Düsseldorf, 9

Easter Rising, 4, 14, 20–1, 23–34, 49, 55, 83, 110, 116; Kathleen Lynn and, 1, 2, 18, 126, 139
Edinburgh, 79
Edinburgh Hospital and Dispensary for Women and Children, 16
education, 1, 3, 8–12, 15, 48, 51, 76, 104
Ely House, 122
'Emergency': see Second World War
Emerson, William, 82
Enright, Margaret, 78–9
Episcopalians: see Church of Ireland
eugenics, 70, 101, 102
Evans, Gladys, 22, 57

Farrell, Isolde, 132
Federation of Irish Industries, 128
feminism, 14, 38, 55, 56, 64, 93, 110, 146, 150
Fermanagh, County, 66
Ferriter, Diarmaid, 42, 107
ffrench-Mullen, Douglas, 75, 84
ffrench-Mullen, Eileen, 75, 88
ffrench-Mullen, Madeleine, 5, 21, 49, 108; and Cumann na dTeachtaire, 35–7, 40; in Easter Rising and aftermath, 23–5, 28–9; relationship between Kathleen Lynn and, 3–4, 21–3, 32, 84, 113, 123, 125; and Rathmines and Rathgar Urban District Council, 52–3; and St Ultan's Hospital, 68–9, 73–5, 77–8, 81, 82
ffrench-Mullen, Pearl, 3
Fianna Fáil, 51, 97, 105, 107–11, 122, 129–30, 136, 152, 156
Finland, 10
Finn, Irene, 2
First World War, 3, 22–3, 28, 42–3, 45, 64, 67, 107, 109, 152
Foley, Brigid, 27
force-feeding of prisoners, 22, 34
France, 64
Franco, Francisco, 109
Freemasonry, 104, 116
Friends of Soviet Russia, 49, 50
Froggatt, Peter, 2
Fullerton, Kathleen Lynn, 1, 4

Gaelic Athletic Association, 73
Gaelic League, 73
Gandhi, M.K. ('Mahatma'), 107
Garvin, Tom, 46
gastroenteritis, 78
German-Irish Society, 132
Germany, 9, 71, 109, 130–2, 149
Gibbons, Mother Columba, 74, 87
Gifford, Sidney, 29
Ginnell, Alice, 35
Glasnevin Cemetery, 43
Glenmalure, 80, 92, 111, 123, 139, 153
Glynn, Sir Joseph, 95
Gonne, Iseult, 61
Gonne, Maud: see under MacBride
Grangegorman, 112
Green, Alice Stopford, 39, 74, 75, 86
Gregory, Lady (Augusta), 112
Griffin, Lucy, 72, 73
Griffith, Arthur, 34, 42, 46
Guinness family, 7–8
Guinness, Sir Arthur (later Lord Ardilaun): see under Ardilaun

Harold's Cross, 70
Hart, Peter, 138
Haslam, Anna, 19, 56
Haslam, Thomas, 19
Hayes, Richard, 39
Hazelwood, 6
health, public: see public health
health committees, 65
Healy, Tim, 47, 111
Herlihy, Donal, 135
Heuston, Sean, 29
Hitler, Adolf, 109, 129–31, 134
Hohenzollern dynasty, 43
Holocaust, 131
Holy Ghost Fathers, 97
Home Rule Bill (1912), 19
housing, 42, 53, 68, 70, 80, 85, 105, 108, 119, 133
Humphreys, Síghle, 28, 49, 138
hunger strikes, 34, 77
Hurley, Ursula, 154–5

illegitimacy, 69, 76, 79, 89
India, 107
industrial schools, 125
Infant Aid Society, 67
infant mortality, 54, 64–9, 76–9, 85–7, 94–5, 108, 113, 124–5, 134
influenza pandemic, 18, 40–5, 73
Inghínidhe na hÉireann, 5, 20
International Red Cross Committee, 48, 77
Inter-State Post-Graduate Assembly, 81
Irish Citizen (newspaper), 38, 56, 150

Irish Citizen Army, 20–1, 23–6, 28, 33, 56, 111, 130, 149
Irish Civil War, 47, 58, 81, 84–5, 132
Irish Free State, 47–8, 50–1, 55, 77, 79, 85–6, 90, 92, 104, 148; Catholic Church and, 114; conservatism dominant in, 2; Protestants in, 147; sectarian divisions in, 97; women in, 155
Irish Guild of SS Luke, Cosmos and Damian, 97
Irish Guild of the Church: see Cumann Gaelach na hEaglaise
Irish Hospitals' Sweepstakes, 95–7, 104, 115
Irish Housewives' Association, 63, 137
Irish language, 74–5, 125–6, 148
Irish Medical Association, 135, 136, 144
Irish National Aid, 23, 33
Irish National Anti-Tuberculosis League, 70, 120–2
Irish Paediatric Club/Association, 98
Irish Press, 48, 110
Irish Red Cross, 121, 122
Irish Republican Army, 97, 108, 109
Irish Republican Prisoners Dependants' Fund, 27
Irish Transport and General Workers Union, 18
Irish Volunteers, 18, 20, 23
Irish War of Independence, 40, 44, 48, 53, 70, 74–5, 81–4, 132, 151
Irish White Cross, 48, 75, 88, 132, 143
Irish Women's Franchise League, 19–20
Irish Women's Reform League, 22
Irish Women's Suffrage and Local Government Association, 19, 37, 56
Irish Women's Suffrage Federation, 18
Irish Women's Workers' Union, 19, 32–3
'Irregulars', 48
Italy, 149

Jackson, Alvin, 23
Jacob, Rosamund, 49, 52, 53
Jacob, Tom, 53
Japan, 130, 151
Jellicoe, Anne, 15, 139
Jesuits, 119, 139
Jews, 109, 130–1
Jex-Blake, Sophia, 10–11, 16–17
Johnson, Stafford, 97, 99, 104, 121–2, 144

Jordan, Donald, 7
Jordan, Nancy, 106
Joyce, William ('Lord Haw Haw'), 129
Juries Act 1927, 84

K Club, 126
Kelly, Adrian, 127
Kennedy, Finola, 98, 137
Keogh, Dermot, 135
Kettle, Mary, 52–4, 138
Kilbride, 83
Kilbrittain, 70
Killala, 6
Killaney, 6
Killybegs, 132
Kilmainham Gaol, 23, 27–30, 48
Kilskyne, 93
King's and Queen's College of Physicians in Ireland, 16
Knights of St Columbanus, 97, 121–2, 137
Knirck, Jason, 46

Ladies' Land League, 7
Laffan, Michael, 26, 33
Lambeth Conference, 93
Land League, 7
Land War, 7, 8
Larkin, Delia, 19
Larkin, James, 18
Lausanne, 47
Lawson, William, 67
League of Women Delegates: see Cumann na dTeachtaire
Lea-Wilson, Marie, 97–8, 115, 116
Lea-Wilson, Percival, 116
Lee, J.J., 2
Lemass, Sean, 108, 130
Lenin, V.I., 49
Lewis, Jane, 81
Liberty Hall, 23, 24, 32
Limerick, 33, 39, 107, 120, 141
Little Mothers' Clubs (US), 82
local government, 37, 73, 115, 127
Local Government Board, 38, 42, 86, 141
Lock Hospital, 38, 69, 80
London, 68, 79
London School of Medicine for Women, 10–11
Longford, County, 7
Lucey, Cornelius, 127–8
Lurgan, 119, 124
Lutherans, 132
Lynn family, 6, 32, 44
Lynn, Alexander, 50
Lynn, Anna, 84, 113
Lynn, Catherine Wynne, 6
Lynn, John, 6, 38, 60, 83–4, 112–13, 136
Lynn, Muriel, 6, 32, 84, 90, 112, 136–7
Lynn, Nan, 6, 31, 83, 84, 112

Lynn, Robert, 6, 7, 31, 36, 44, 83
Lynn, Winsome, 136, 144
Lynn House, 1, 146
Lyons, J.B., 2

Macardle, Dorothy, 48, 111, 113
MacBride, John, 61
MacBride, Maud Gonne, 20, 34, 61, 74, 111, 135
MacBride, Sean, 135
McCabe, Anna, 125
McCourt, Frank, 141
MacCurtain, Margaret, 50
MacDonagh, Thomas, 29
McElligott, T.J., 123–4
MacEntee, Seán, 127
McGloughlin, Stephen, 128
McIlroy, Louise, 103
McPolin, James, 107, 120
McQuaid, Archbishop John Charles, 93, 97, 103–4, 114, 120–2, 125, 127, 136
McQuaide, Bessie, 6
MacSwiney, Mary, 46, 48
MacSwiney, Terence, 77
McTier, Martha, 148–9
McWhorter, Mary, 77
Magill, Isabel, 76
Maguire, Conor, 122
Maguire, Katherine, 9, 10, 19, 20, 22, 66, 69–71
Mahon, Bríd, 112
Mallin, Michael, 29
malnutrition, 65, 106, 123, 124, 128
Manchester, 9, 68, 72
Manchester Babies' Hospital, 43
Manchester High School for Girls, 43
Manchester Infant Hospital, 76–7
Mansion House, 34, 38, 39, 44, 46, 50, 110, 123
Marie Stopes Clinic, 101
Markievicz, Constance, 20, 21, 24, 27–9, 33–5, 40, 146
Mater Misericordiae Hospital, Belfast, 120
Mater Misericordiae Hospital, Dublin, 34, 68
Maternity and Child Welfare Scheme (Dublin), 135
Maxwell, Anne: see under Wynne
Mayo, Charles, 90
Mayo, County, 1, 6–7, 44, 93, 154
Mayo Clinic, 90
Meath, County, 69, 83, 87, 93
Meath Hospital, 137, 144
Medical Council of Ireland, 1, 146
Meenan, F.O.C., 11
midwifery, 11, 71
Mitchell, David, 11
Mitchell, Margaret, 124

Index

Mitchell, Susan, 21, 57
Molony, Helena ('Emer'), 2, 20, 23, 25, 27–8, 30, 34–5, 40, 49, 78, 123
Montessori, Maria, 93, 106, 155
Moorhead, T.G., 101–4, 138
Morash, Christopher, 49
mortality rates, 15, 54, 64–9, 76–9, 85–7, 94–5, 108, 113, 124–5, 133–4
Mother and Child Scheme, 134–6, 144
motherhood, 64, 65, 76, 80–1, 92, 106, 149
Mountjoy Prison, 29–31, 34
Mount Sinai Hospital, New York, 82
Mullaghfarry, 6
Mulvany, Isabella, 9
Murphy, Kathleen, 132
Mussolini, Benito, 109

National Archives of Ireland, 62
National Association for Promoting the Medical Education of Women, 17
National Association for Women's Suffrage, 65
National BCG Centre, 119, 134
National Children's Hospital, 5, 78, 93, 95, 97–105
nationalism, Irish, 2, 4, 12, 14, 20, 22, 23, 29
National League of Health, 53
National Maternity Hospital, 11
National Museum of Ireland, 57, 130, 139, 145
National University of Ireland, 97, 104
National University Women Graduates' Association, 2
Nesbitt, George, 45
Newcastle, 66
Newgrange, 69
Newman, John Henry, 100
New York City, 82, 96
New Zealand, 67
Nic Dhonnchadha, Lil, 126, 156
North Dublin Union, 49
Northern Ireland, 47, 48, 79, 84, 131
Norway, 10
Notification of Births Acts, 65, 66
Novick, Ben, 38
Nugent family, 138
Nugent, Susie, 111
nurses and nursing, 68, 72, 84, 88, 110, 122, 156
nutrition, 106, 124, 125

O'Brennan, Kathleen, 48
O'Brien, Kathleen Cruise, 49
O'Brien, Nora Connolly, 25–6, 84
O'Brien-Kennedy, Francis, 93

O'Casey, Sean, 21, 49
O'Connor, Rory, 75
O'Dea, Jimmy, 112
O'Doherty, Rose, 127, 155
O'Donnell, Frank Hugh, 15
O'Donnell, Peadar, 49, 152
O'Donovan, J.M., 121
O'Duffy, Eoin, 109
O'Farrelly, Agnes, 39
O'Higgins, Kevin, 47
O'Kelly, Sean T., 97, 129
Old ICA Association, 111
'Operation Shamrock', 132
Our Lady's Hospital for Sick Children, 114, 136
Ovenden, Isabella, 9

pacifism, 2
paediatrics, 1, 2, 10, 14, 73, 88, 94, 101–2, 125, 154
Paine, Thomas, 154
Palmer, Marguerite, 22
Pankhurst, Sylvia, 4, 19, 20, 56
Parnell, Charles Stewart, 47
Pašeta, Senia, 12
Paul, St, 146
Peamount Sanatorium, 66, 70, 121
Pearse, Pádraig, 23, 49, 74, 77, 139
Pearse, William, 23
Pembroke Urban District Council, 65
Pentonville Prison, London, 60
Perolz, Marie, 27
philanthropy: see charitable activities
Plunket Society, 67
Plunkett family, 14
Plunkett, Fiona, Countess, 30, 35, 36, 38
Plunkett, George Noble, Count, 34, 152
Plunkett, Grace, 29
Plunkett, Joseph, 29
Poor Clare Orphanage, Cavan, 127
Poor Law Guardians, 65, 73, 85
Post-Sanatorium League, 120
poverty and the poor, 1, 2, 105, 123, 125, 128, 133, 139, 150; in Dublin, 15, 21, 67–8, 84, 98, 103, 119, 126, 143; in Limerick, 141; in County Mayo, 6, 7
Powell, Malachy, 133
Power, Eileen, 14, 147
Power, Jennie Wyse, 19, 32, 35, 39
Price, Dorothy Stopford, 71, 74, 99, 102, 116, 121–2, 128, 133–4, 139, 147, 154
Prisoners (Temporary Discharge for Ill Health) Act (1913): see Cat and Mouse Act

prisons and prisoners, 22, 26–32, 34, 42, 47–8, 55, 107, 109, 129, 131
Prosser, Georgina, 14
prostitution, 37, 38
Protestants and Protestantism, 8–9, 14, 93–4, 97, 102, 120, 125, 137, 147
public health, 37–40, 42, 53, 64–7, 73, 106, 119, 124, 135
Public Health Act (Ireland), 59

Quakers, 19, 132

Radical Club, 49, 50
Rathdown Union, 72
Rathmines, 1, 14, 20, 33, 41, 113, 146
Rathmines and Pembroke Joint Hospital Board, 53
Rathmines and Rathgar Urban District Council, 52, 53, 54, 63
Red Cross: see under American; International; Irish
religious orders, 85, 122
Representation of the People Act (1918), 37
republicans and republicanism, 32, 116; and Irish Free State, 47–50, 152; Kathleen Lynn and, 1–2, 4, 18, 20, 25, 27–9, 33–4, 37, 41, 52, 70, 107–10, 126, 129, 138, 145; and St Ultan's Hospital, 75, 77, 115; and United States, 31, 45–6, 82; women and, 46, 138, 145
Richmond Barracks, 27, 28
Richmond Lunatic Asylum, 11
rickets, 71
Rockefeller Foundation, 81, 96
Rossclare, 66
Rotunda Lying-In Hospital, 11, 13, 134
Royal College of Physicians and Surgeons of Glasgow, 70
Royal College of Physicians of Ireland, 4, 5, 17
Royal College of Science, 10
Royal College of Surgeons in Ireland, 12, 13, 16, 133
Royal Free Hospital, London, 103
Royal Institute of Public Health, 66
Royal University of Ireland, 12, 55, 71
Royal Victoria Eye and Ear Hospital, 11, 13, 14, 31
Russell, George, 74
Russell, M.J., 85
Russell, Matthew, 81
Ryan, Frank, 49
Ryan, Louise, 48
Ryan, Phyllis, 129

St Andrews, University of, 16
St Ann's Church, 46
St Catherine's School and Orphanage, 70
St Enda's School, 23, 74
St Mary's Home, Ballsbridge, 139, 154
St Michael's Convent, Navan, 74
St Ultan's Hospital for Infants, 1–2, 10, 16, 31, 39, 42–3, 53–6, 63–4, 81, 88, 93, 115, 125, 145; board of, 127; establishment of, 68–9, 72–3; funding of, 74–5, 77, 82, 113; and housing, 80; infant mortality at, 67, 78–9, 95; Kathleen Lynn and, 85, 149–50, 154; motherhood training at, 76–7; proposed merger between National Children's Hospital and, 93, 95, 97–105; nurses at, 72, 84, 110; rates of pay at, 153; treatment of tuberculosis at, 119, 128, 133–4; woman doctors at, 66–7, 70–2
St Ultan's Hospital Utility Society, 80, 105
St Vincent's Hospital, 68
Samaritans, 155
San Francisco, 74, 75
sanitation movement, 65
Save the German Children Society, 132, 138
Scandinavian Women's Sanitary Association, 65
school meals, 54, 63, 107, 137
Scott, Michael, 95, 98, 112, 128
Second World War, 105, 119, 125, 129–30, 133, 139, 152
'separation women', 28
Sheehy, David, 92
Sheehy Skeffington, Andrée, 111
Sheehy Skeffington, Hanna, 3, 19–20, 22, 23, 49, 52, 53, 63, 111
Sheridan, John D., 151
Ship Street Barracks, 26–7, 30
Shrule, 7
Sinn Féin, 3, 19, 34–40, 42–5, 48–55, 58–9, 64, 69, 108, 111, 129, 148–50
Sinn Féin League of Women Delegates: see Cumann na dTeachtaire
Sir Patrick Dun's Hospital, 13, 72
Sisters of Mercy, 122
Six Counties: see Northern Ireland
Sláinte (journal), 67
Sláinte na nGaedheal, 72
Slane, 69
Sligo, County, 6

smallpox, 107
Smartt, Francis, 7, 16
Smith, Anna, 96
Smith, Trevor, 98
Smyly Homes, 102
socialism, 2, 18, 25–6, 49, 93, 107, 121, 145, 150, 152
Solomons, Bethel, 109
'souperism', 102
South America, 75
Soviet Union, 49, 107, 109, 130, 131
Spanish Civil War, 109
spirituality, 8, 33, 82–3, 130, 151–2
Stack, Austin, 46
Stack, Nora, 98
Stanford, W.B., 147
Statistical and Social Inquiry Society of Ireland, 124
sterilisation, 101, 102
Stillorgan Children's Sunshine Home, 71
Stokes, Barbara, 155
Stradbrook Hall, 3
Strangman, Mary, 22
suffragism, 1, 12, 18–23, 37, 47, 55–6, 69
Sweden, 134
Switzerland, 47, 48

Tallaght Hospital, 5
Teach Ultáin: see under St Ultan's
Te Brake, Janet, 7
tenant farmers, 7, 8
Tennant, Elizabeth, 19, 70–1, 79, 95, 99
Tipperary, 47, 97
Tone, Theobald Wolfe, 1–2, 33–4, 51–2, 130, 139, 145
Trinity College, Dublin, 10, 66, 71, 93–4, 96–7, 101–2, 128, 137, 139
tuberculosis, 66, 70, 76, 94, 105, 112, 116, 119–22, 128, 133, 136
Tweedy, Hilda, 137
typhus, 117

Ultan, St, 69, 87, 156
unionism, 1, 32, 90
United Irishmen, 148–50
United States, 13, 31, 45–6, 48, 74, 81–2, 105, 113, 131, 148
universities, 9, 10, 12
University College, Cork, 78, 121
University College, Dublin, 96, 106, 128; Medical School, 10–13
utility societies, 80

vaccination, 65, 94, 107, 133–4
venereal diseases, 37–40, 42, 59, 69, 72, 73, 80
Versailles, Treaty of, 45
Volunteer Dependants' Fund, 33

Wales, Albert Edward, Prince of: see under Albert
Walsh, Archbishop William, 45, 73
Warrenpoint, 112, 136
water supply, 141
Waterford, 47
Webb, Deborah, 54, 63, 87–8
Webb, Ella, 22, 66–7, 71–2, 98, 99
Webb, George, 71
Whelan, James, 111
White, Jack, 93–4
Wicklow, County, 9, 33, 80, 111, 112, 138, 147
widows and orphans' pensions, 52, 63
Wilson, Adrian, 7
women: and Anglo-Irish Treaty, 46; and child care, 122; James Connolly on, 21, 56; Constitution and, 110–11; and education, 1, 11, 12, 15, 76; with large families, 2; and health, 64–6; in Irish Citizen Army, 24, 25; in Irish Free State, 4, 92, 155; and Land League, 7, 8; Kathleen Lynn on, 44; and medicine, 9–13, 19, 68, 148; position of, 147; as prisoners, 22, 26–31, 48; and Irish republicanism, 138; and Sinn Féin, 34–8, 54, 55, 69; socialism and, 145; and suffragism, 18; in universities, 9, 10, 12; working hours of, 108
Women Prisoners' Defence Association, 48
Women's Education League of San Francisco, 74
Women's National Health Association, 65–7, 70, 71, 121
Women's Sanitary Organisation, 65
Women's Social and Political Union, 19, 22
working class, 56, 124, 127, 135
Wynne family, 6, 9
Wynne, Anne Maxwell, 6
Wynne, Catherine: see under Lynn
Wynne, Florence, 36, 44, 84, 123
Wynne, Owen, 6
Wynne, Richard, 6
Wynne, William, 4, 90, 123, 155

Yeats, Jack B., 74
Young, Bishop Matthew, 130, 139, 145

Zürich, 111–12